UNLOCKING THE POWER OF THE BRAIN WITH NEUROBIOLOGY: UNDERSTANDING BRAIN FUNCTIONS AND LEARNING MECHANISMS

D. Beck

Cover design by: Art Painter
Library of Congress Control Number: 2018675309
Printed in the United States of America

I Want to thank you and congratulate you for buying my book
Unlocking the Power of the Brain
with Neurobiology

CONTENTS

INTODUCTION

Neurobiology is the study of the structure and function of the nervous system, which includes the brain, spinal cord, and peripheral nerves. Neurobiologists investigate how these organs interact to process information from our environment, regulate behaviour and emotions, and control conscious thought. They also examine how neurological diseases such as Alzheimer's or Parkinson's affect different parts of the nervous system.

Neurobiologists use a variety of tools and techniques to investigate the brain such as electrophysiology, optogenetics, neuroimaging, and behavioural experiments. By combining these approaches with functional genomics, they can gain insight into how different areas of the brain are connected and interact.

Advances in neuroscience have led to the development of treatments such as deep brain stimulation and genetic therapies, which can help improve symptoms associated with neurological disorders. Neurobiology also has implications for understanding how our environment affects us and developing new strategies to prevent or reduce the risk of neurological diseases. Research in this field is ongoing as scientists work to uncover the mysteries of the brain.

Ultimately, neurobiologists seek to gain a better understanding of the mind and how it works, so that we can discover more effective treatments for neurological disorders. Progress in this field will likely have far-reaching implications for our health and well-being. As such, neurobiology research will continue to play an important role in advancing medical science. It may even provide us with insight into the origins of consciousness and how we perceive and interact with our environment. With a better understanding of the brain, neurobiologists will be able to continue to shape medical science for years to come.

Neurobiology can also help us gain insight into other areas such as behavioural economics and human decision-making. By studying how neuronal networks and pathways influence our behaviour, neurobiologists can gain an understanding of what causes us to make certain choices and how our environment affects these decisions. This could allow us to develop more effective interventions for tackling addiction or mental illness. Neurobiology research may also help us understand why some people are better able to cope with stress, while others are more prone to anxiety or depression.

Hello, it's me, D.Beck . Before you start reading my book I would like to ask you a favor: If you enjoy reading the book can you please leave an honest review for me in Amazon? - it will mean a lot to me! Thanks in advantage, and now be ready to learn how to understan the mind and how it works :)

CHAPTER 1: ABOUT NEUROBIOLOGY

W hat is neurobiological?
Neurobiology is a branch of biology that focuses on the study of how the nervous system works. It involves examining the structure and function of neurons, which are cells responsible for the transmission of information throughout our body. Neurobiology also examines how neurons interact to create complex behaviour in humans, animals, and plants.

Researchers use neurobiological principles to explore various topics including brain development, memory formation, learning and behaviour, and neurological diseases. By understanding how the nervous system works, we can better understand how to treat conditions or disorders affecting the brain or nervous system.

This field of study has become increasingly important with the advancement of modern technology. Scientists are now able to use sophisticated imaging techniques such as fMRI and PET scans to explore the activity of neurons in our brains. This has allowed researchers to gain a better understanding of how the brain works and how it affects different aspects of our lives.

Understanding neurobiology is key to unlocking the mysteries of the human brain, which can lead to advances in medicine, psychology, and other sciences. With more research, we can even come to a better understanding of how the brain works and why it behaves in certain ways. Neurobiology is an ever-evolving field, one that will continue to offer fascinating insights into the workings of the human brain for many years to come.

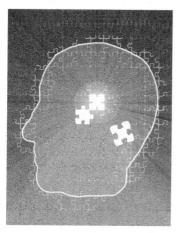

By studying neurobiology, scientists hope to gain insight into neurological diseases and conditions such as Alzheimer's, Parkinson's, multiple sclerosis, and traumatic brain injury. This can lead to improved diagnosis and treatments for these conditions, as well as a better understanding of the relationship between our bodies and brains. Neurobiology is an incredibly important field of study that will continue to expand our knowledge about the human brain.

With increased knowledge and research in this field comes new opportunities for further exploration. For example, scientists are now able to use brain imaging to study the effects of different drugs on the brain, as well as explore how certain neurological conditions can be treated with medication. This research could potentially lead to new treatments and cures for debilitating diseases like Alzheimer's or Parkinson's.

History Of Neurobiology

The history of Neurobiology can be traced back to ancient times when it was believed that the brain was the seat of consciousness and emotion. In 551 BC, the Indian philosopher-surgeon Sushruta described the anatomy of the nervous system in his treatise Sushruta Samhita. He noted that nerve fibres were associated with particular organs and senses, and proposed that there was a link between the nervous system and intelligence.

In the 4th century BC, Hippocrates theorized that physical diseases had psychological causes and effects. He suggested that mental illnesses could be treated with a combination of diet, exercise, drugs, and other therapies. In subsequent centuries, scientific understanding of the brain increased as philosophers and physicians explored the relationship between mind and body.

In the 17th century, Thomas Willis wrote extensively about the structure and anatomy of the brain in his book Cerebri Anatomy. His work was influential in establishing a view of the brain as having physical components that interacted with each other to produce behaviour. In 1793,

Italian physician Luigi Galvani discovered[1] that electricity could be used to stimulate muscles, giving rise to neurophysiology.

The 19th century saw a rapid expansion of knowledge about the brain, as scientists such as Georges Gilles de la Tourette and Jean-Martin Charcot studied mental illness and neurology respectively. In 1891, Ivan Pavlov discovered the conditioning reflex in dogs, laying the groundwork for the field of behavioural neuroscience. By the early 20th century, scientists had established a strong link between brain function and behaviour, paving the way for modern Neurobiology.

Today, Neurobiology remains an important and growing field of study. Scientists continue to explore how different parts of the brain interact with each other to produce complex behaviours, while technological advances in imaging technology and computing have enabled a greater understanding of the brain's anatomy and function. With more research, Neurobiology has the potential to deepen our understanding of the human mind and its connection to physical health, mental health, and behaviour.

Explain Key Concepts And Terminology

At its core, neurobiology focuses on understanding the physiology of the brain and understanding how each component in the nervous system interacts with one another. In order to achieve this, neurobiologists must be familiar with the anatomy and physiology of the nervous system, along with molecular biology, biochemistry, genetics, and pharmacology.

Neurobiology has several key concepts that need to be understood in order to study the brain effectively. Neurons are cells that form connections between the brain and other parts of the body. These neurons communicate with each other through electrical signals known as action potentials. Synapses are the sites where neurons interact and form connections, and neurotransmitters are chemicals that allow neurons to pass information between one another. Neurotransmitters can also modulate the activity of certain neurons, which allows for more complex behaviours like learning and memory formation.

In addition to understanding key concepts, neurobiologists must be familiar with various terms used when talking about the brain. The most common term is 'neuroplasticity', which refers to the ability of the brain to adapt and change over time in response to new experiences. Other important terms include 'dendritic spines', 'axons', 'synapses', and 'neurotransmitters'. Lastly, neurobiologists should be familiar with brain imaging techniques such as magnetic resonance imaging (MRI) and functional magnetic resonance imaging (fMRI). These are used to study the structure of the brain and how it functions in response to different tasks.

What Is The Difference Between Neurobiology And Neuroscience?

Neurobiology is the study of cells and molecules that make up the nervous system, while neuroscience focuses on the structure and function of the nervous system. Neurobiology examines how neurons interact with each other to form networks that carry out various functions. Neuroscience focuses on understanding how these networks contribute to behaviour, emotion, cognition, and sensory processes. Both fields involve research into anatomy and physiology, but neurobiology is more focused on the molecular and cellular levels. Neurobiology studies how nerve cells communicate with each other through chemical signals, whereas neuroscience looks at how these signals are integrated into higher-level processes such as memory, language, perception, and emotion. Both disciplines look at how neural networks influence behaviour and cognition, but neurobiology takes a more detailed approach by studying the workings of individual cells.

In addition, neurobiology also looks at how genetic and environmental factors can affect the structure and function of neurons. For example, researchers may examine how certain mutations in genes that code for proteins involved in nerve communication can cause neurological disorders. On the other hand, neuroscience focuses on understanding how these networks interact with each other to influence behaviour, thought processes, and emotions. For instance, researchers may investigate how different regions of the brain interact to produce our conscious experience.

Ultimately both neuroscience and neurobiology are important tools for understanding how the brain functions and contributes to behaviour. Neurobiology looks at individual cells and molecules while neuroscience focuses on larger networks of neurons. By combining these two disciplines, researchers can gain a deeper understanding of how the brain works.

Other closely related fields to neuroscience and neurobiology include psychology, cognitive science, and philosophy. Psychology focuses on understanding human behavior while cognitive science examines how information is processed in the mind. Philosophy looks at issues such as consciousness, free will, and ethics. These disciplines often overlap with neuroscience and neurobiology in their studies of the brain. By combining knowledge from all fields, researchers can gain a more thorough understanding of the human mind and its complexities.

The advancements in neuroscience and neurobiology have enabled us to better understand how the brain works, what roles different parts play, and how these processes affect our lives. From treating mental illnesses to creating new technologies that use neural networks to improve accuracy and speed, understanding the brain is essential for advancing our knowledge of the human condition.

Overall, neurobiology and neuroscience are both fascinating fields that allow us to gain insight into how the brain works at different levels. By studying individual cells as well as larger networks of neurons, scientists can uncover new insights about how our brains work and how this affects behaviour.

How Does Neurobiology Work?

Neurobiology is a branch of biology that studies the structure and function of the nervous system, as well as how it relates to behaviour. Neurobiologists focus on understanding how nerve cells, or neurons, transmit information from one part of the body to another. They also study how this information is processed in order for us to feel, think, and act.

Neurons are complex cells that contain multiple parts, including cell bodies, dendrites, and axons. Cell bodies are the main components of neurons and contain organelles like mitochondria and nuclei. Dendrites branch out from the cell body in order to transmit electrical signals to other cells. The axon is a long nerve fibre that carries electrical signals away from the cell body and can be up to a meter long in humans.

Neurobiologists study how neurons communicate with each other. Electrical signals are sent from one neuron to another through structures called synapses. When the signal reaches the synaptic terminal of one neuron, chemicals called neurotransmitters are released into the gap between the two neurons, causing a change in the electrical charge of the receiving neuron. This process is repeated until the signal reaches its intended destination.

In addition to studying neurons, neurobiologists also study how certain areas of the brain interact with each other and how those interactions can influence behaviour. For example, they may investigate how different regions work together to regulate appetite or control emotions. Neurobiologists use a variety of tools to study the brain, including imaging techniques like magnetic resonance imaging (MRI) and computed tomography (CT).

How Does Neurobiology Affect Behavior?

Neurobiological processes are involved in every aspect of behaviour, from mood and emotion to movement and memory.

The brain has three main parts: the cerebrum (the largest part), the cerebellum (a smaller part that coordinates movement), and the brainstem (which connects the brain to the spinal cord and controls basic functions like breathing, heart rate, and digestion).

Each of these parts has its own set of neurons that help carry out specific tasks. For example, the cerebrum is responsible for higher-level processing, such as decision-making and problem-solving. The cerebellum helps with coordination and movement. And the brainstem is responsible for basic functions like breathing and heart rate.

Neurons also play a role in emotion and mood by releasing neurotransmitters, such as serotonin, dopamine, and norepinephrine, which can affect our behaviour. Neurotransmitters also help us learn new information and form memories.

Finally, hormones like cortisol are released in response to stress and can affect our behaviour. Hormones can also play a role in appetite, sleep patterns, and emotional regulation.

Breakthrough Discoveries In Neurological Disorders

Recent advances in the field of neurobiology have made it possible to gain a greater understanding of neurological disorders and their potential treatments. This has led to breakthroughs in the diagnosis and treatment of neurological disorders, such as Parkinson's disease, Alzheimer's disease, Multiple Sclerosis, Huntington's disease, Amyotrophic Lateral Sclerosis (ALS), Tourette

Syndrome and Autism Spectrum Disorder.

Researchers have identified various genetic mutations that contribute to the development of these disorders, allowing for earlier diagnosis and tailored treatments. For example, a mutation in the LRRK2 gene has been linked to an increased risk of developing Parkinson's disease, while mutations in the genes DISC1 and CNTNAP2 are associated with an increased risk for autism spectrum disorder.

In addition to genetic factors, environmental and lifestyle factors have also been identified as potential contributors to the development of neurological disorders. Studies have shown that exposure to certain toxins such as lead, mercury, and DDT can increase the risk of developing Parkinson's disease, while air pollution has been linked to an increased risk for Alzheimer's disease. Other lifestyle factors, such as diet and exercise, are also associated with an increased risk of developing certain neurological disorders.

The development of new treatments has been greatly aided by advances in brain imaging technology, which allows researchers to identify changes in the brain that can be linked to different neurological disorders. For example, magnetic resonance imaging (MRI) is used to detect changes in the structure or metabolism of brain tissue associated with disorders like Alzheimer's, while positron emission tomography (PET) can identify changes in the activity of certain brain regions that are linked to conditions such as Parkinson's.

Importance Of Studying Neurobiology

Studying neurobiology is of great importance in the medical field due to its potential to help us understand and treat neurological disorders. Neurobiology research has lead to a better understanding of the brain and how it functions, as well as disease processes connected with neurological conditions. This knowledge can be used to develop treatments that target specific areas or processes within the brain, such as those involved in learning and memory, motor control, or emotional regulation. Additionally, it can be used to develop interventions, such as medications and medical devices, that help improve the lives of people with neurological disorders.

Moreover, neurobiology is essential for understanding how different environmental factors can affect our behaviour and mental health. Studies have shown that exposure to toxins or pollutants can alter brain development and lead to cognitive impairment or mental health issues. Understanding how these environmental factors interact with the brain can help inform prevention measures that protect our mental and physical well-being.

In sum, neurobiology has the potential to

revolutionize medicine by providing insight into various neurological disorders, as well as how the environment impacts our brains in order to promote healthy living. As such, research in this field should be encouraged and supported to improve our quality of life.

Finally, studying neurobiology can also help us understand the mystery of consciousness - how we perceive the world and how our brains work to give rise to it. Understanding this complex phenomenon could lead to new ways of treating or even preventing certain neurological disorders, as well as providing insight into why some people are more prone to developing psychological disorders. This knowledge could provide invaluable tools for healthcare professionals and help improve the lives of those affected by neurological conditions.

The potential of neurobiology is immense, and with further research, it can become a powerful tool in medicine and psychology. We must invest in this field so that we can understand how our brains work and develop treatments that improve the lives of those affected by neurological disorders.

CHAPTER 2: UNDERSTANDING THE BASIC STRUCTURE AND FUNCTION OF NEURONS

Neurons are highly specialized cells that use electrical and chemical signals to communicate. Each neuron has three main parts: a cell body, dendrites, and an axon.

A cell body is the central region of a neuron which contains most of its metabolic machinery. This provides energy to help maintain active neurons, as well as synthesize and store neurotransmitters. The cell body also contains other organelles such as mitochondria, Golgi bodies, and endoplasmic reticulum. Additionally, it serves as the main hub for incoming macromolecules or ions to be used in the neuron's metabolic processes. The nucleus, which contains genetic material, is also found within the cell body.

Dendrites are an essential component of neurons, which play a crucial role in the communication of information within the nervous system. These tree-like extensions emanate from the neuron's cell body and function to receive signals from other neurons. Each dendrite forms numerous synapses with other neurons, allowing them to transmit incoming electrical signals towards the cell body. This complex network of connections enables the intricate and rapid communication that underlies our every thought, action, and sensation.

The axon is another key part of a neuron. This long, slender projection conducts electrical impulses away from the neuron's cell body. Its primary function is to transmit information to different neurons, muscles, and glands. In some cases, axons can be quite short, while in others they can be a meter or more long. The axon ends in multiple growths known as axon terminals which are used to send signals to other neurons. To speed up the transmission of the electrical signal, the axon is often covered in a layer of fatty tissue called the myelin sheath. This sheath functions much like the insulation around an electrical wire, reducing the signal's loss and increasing the speed at which it travels.

Role Of Neurotransmitters In Neuronal Communication

Neurons communicate with one another by releasing chemical signals known as neurotransmitters. When the electrical signal reaches the end of the neuron, it triggers the release of a neurotransmitter from special structures at the end called synaptic vesicles. The released neurotransmitter then binds to specific receptor sites on receptors located on another neuron's membrane. This binding activates or inactivates the postsynaptic neuron, depending on the type of neurotransmitter and its receptors. By sending these chemical signals down a chain of neurons, messages are passed between different parts of the body. Neurotransmitters can also have effects on muscles or glands to control movement and secretions. Examples of common neurotransmitters include dopamine, serotonin, acetylcholine, norepinephrine, and glutamate.

Dopamine, a type of neurotransmitter, plays a crucial role in how we perceive pleasure and reward. It is extensively involved in various brain functions such as learning, motivation, attention, and mood. When an action leads to a reward, it is the dopamine system that reinforces this positive outcome, encouraging the behaviour to be repeated. Moreover, dopamine is critical in motor control and its deficiency is linked to serious neurological conditions such as Parkinson's disease. By understanding the function and influence of dopamine, we gain profound insights into human behaviour, psychology, and certain pathologies.

Serotonin, another neurotransmitter, is predominantly involved in regulating mood, social behaviour, appetite and digestion, sleep, memory, and sexual desire. This neurotransmitter contributes to a feeling of well-being and happiness. It helps regulate the body's sleep-wake cycles and the internal clock. An imbalance in serotonin levels may influence mood in a way that leads to depression. Certain medications, such as selective serotonin reuptake inhibitors (SSRIs), are used to regulate serotonin levels in the brain to treat depression, anxiety, and panic disorders. Understanding serotonin's function and its role in the brain helps deepen our knowledge of mental health conditions and their treatment.

Acetylcholine, yet another crucial neurotransmitter, has manifold roles in the body and brain. In the brain, it plays an important part in attention, learning, and memory. In the rest of the body, acetylcholine acts at neuromuscular junctions to influence muscle contraction and heart rate, and it is involved in transmitting signals in the autonomic nervous system, which regulates functions like digestion and salivation. Notably, a decline in acetylcholine function is associated with memory deficits observed in Alzheimer's disease, further underscoring its importance in cognitive function. Understanding the function and implications of acetylcholine can provide deeper insight into various neurological and physiological processes.

Norepinephrine, another significant neurotransmitter, operates as a vital chemical messenger in the central and peripheral nervous systems. In the brain, norepinephrine is involved in responses to stress and panic, attention, and the control of sleep and arousal. It functions to increase heart rate and blood pumping from the heart. It also increases blood pressure and helps break down fat and increases blood sugar levels to provide more energy to the body. Additionally, norepinephrine plays an important role in mood regulation, and imbalances in this neurotransmitter have been linked to mood disorders such as depression and bipolar disorder. Understanding the role and interaction of norepinephrine in our nervous system can enhance our comprehension of the human response to stress and the underlying mechanisms of mood disorders.

Glutamate, the last neurotransmitter in this discussion but by no means the least, is the most abundant excitatory neurotransmitter in the nervous system. It plays an essential role in normal brain function and is critical for learning, memory formation, and synaptic plasticity, which is the ability of synapses to strengthen or weaken over time, in response to increases or decreases in their activity. Additionally, glutamate is involved in the proliferation and migration of neural progenitor cells, playing a significant part in brain development. On the flip side, excessive amounts of glutamate can lead to excitotoxicity, a process that damages and can ultimately kill neurons. This plays a significant role in many neurological disorders, such as Alzheimer's disease, stroke, and epilepsy. Understanding the role and regulation of glutamate in the brain provides key insights into the functioning of the brain and associated pathologies.

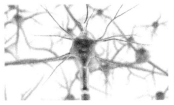

Neurons From Molecules

At the most basic level, neurons are composed of molecules such as proteins and lipids. Proteins act as molecular scaffolding within the neuron, providing structure and binding sites for other proteins and molecules to interact with. Lipids provide insulation to maintain the electrical potential within the neuron while also facilitating communication between different parts of the cell.

Proteins, lipids and other molecules interact to form cell membranes that are essential for neuron functioning. Cell membranes act as a barrier between the inside of the cell and its environment, allowing ions such as potassium, sodium and calcium to enter or exit the neuron depending on their concentration gradients. This process of ion exchange is what generates electrical potentials within neurons.

The flow of ions across the cell membrane also causes small changes in the electrical potential, which can be measured by electrodes placed near the neuron's surface. This type of measurement is called electrophysiology and provides insight into a neuron's behaviour.

Beyond molecules, neurons are composed of organelles that provide structure and guidance to the cell. The nucleus is responsible for storing genetic information and providing instructions for protein synthesis, while mitochondria act as the cell's energy source. Other organelles such as the endoplasmic reticulum help with important processes such as transporting proteins and other molecules within the neuron.

It is the intricate combination of molecules and organelles that allows neurons to be responsible for processing, storing, and transferring information. This is why it is so important to understand the basic structure and function of neurons, as it helps us better understand how our brains work.

Relevance Of Neurobiology In Understanding Human Behaviour

Neuroscience has been an invaluable resource in understanding various aspects of human behaviour. The work conducted by neuroscientists helps us to understand complex neural networks and the role they play in determining our actions and thoughts. By examining the structure of neurons, scientists are able to identify the areas responsible for certain behaviours or mental processes, such as memory formation, motor control, and decision-making.

Additionally, the study of neurons and their development has revealed information about sensory processing, language development, and perceptual processes. This knowledge is highly relevant for psychologists who use it to explain various aspects of human behaviour, such as personality traits or cognitive deficits.

Furthermore, advancements in neurobiology have allowed researchers to gain insight into the role that neural networks play in psychological disorders, such as schizophrenia and dyslexia. By studying the brain structures of those with these conditions, scientists are able to better understand how they affect behaviour and cognition. This not only enables them to develop more effective treatments but also gives them a greater understanding of normal brain functioning.

Neurobiology continues to be an invaluable tool for both clinicians and researchers, offering valuable insights into the complexities of the error occurred during generation. Please try again or contact support if it continues. the human brain and its impact on behaviour. It is an ever-evolving field that continues to provide us with new and exciting discoveries about the inner workings of our minds.

Implications For Medical Treatments

The study of neurobiology also has important implications for medical treatments. By understanding how neurons function, researchers have been able to develop therapies that target certain areas of the brain. For example, deep brain stimulation (DBS) is a technique used to treat certain neurological disorders. In this technique, electrodes are implanted in specific regions of the brain and then used to deliver electrical pulses which stimulate those neurons directly.

This technique has been useful for treating movement disorders such as Parkinson's disease, depression, and obsessive-compulsive disorder. Additionally, it has been used to help reduce pain and improve motor control in patients with neuromuscular disorders.

Neurobiology is also relevant for the treatment of degenerative diseases such as Alzheimer's and Parkinson's. By understanding how neurons communicate and interact with one another, researchers are able to develop drugs that can help slow down or even halt the progression of these diseases.

Overall, the study of neurobiology has tremendous implications for medical treatments and can help us to develop therapies that target specific areas of the brain in order to improve patient outcomes. Neurobiology is a rapidly advancing field with exciting potential for improving human health and well-being.

CHAPTER 3: KEY CONCEPTS
IN NEUROBIOLOGY

Neuronal signalling

Neuronal signalling is the process by which neurons communicate with each other to relay information. It involves the release of neurotransmitters, such as dopamine and serotonin, across synapses that facilitate communication between two cells. Signal transduction is a related concept that occurs when these released neurotransmitters interact with receptors on the post-synaptic neuron, triggering a cascade of molecular changes within it. These changes can ultimately result in the modulation of neuron activity or even death.

The study of neuronal signalling has been instrumental in uncovering many mysteries surrounding the nervous system, including such topics as signal recognition and transduction pathways, axon guidance and plasticity. In recent years, techniques such as optogenetics have allowed researchers to gain unprecedented control over neurons by manipulating their activity with light. This has opened up a world of possibilities in terms of understanding the role of neuronal signalling in various neurological disorders such as Parkinson's and Alzheimer's disease, as well as psychiatric conditions like depression.

In addition to its importance for neuroscience research, neuronal signalling is also an area of great promise for medical treatments. For example, drugs that target neurotransmitters may be used to treat conditions such as depression and anxiety, while newer treatments that use optogenetics could help restore lost motor and cognitive function in patients with neurological disorders. Ultimately, the ability to precisely control neuronal signalling holds great potential for improving the lives of those affected by these devastating diseases.

The field of neuronal signalling is complex and ever-evolving, with a wide range of implications for health and medicine. It is also an area of great potential for further research and development, and its future progress will undoubtedly provide valuable insights into the inner workings of the human brain. With advances in technology and understanding, there is no limit to what we can learn about how neurons communicate.

Neurogenesis

Neurogenesis is the process of generating neurons from stem cells. This process is essential for the development and maintenance of the nervous system, as well as providing repair and regeneration potential. During development, neurogenesis occurs in two distinct periods:

during embryonic development and during adulthood. During embryonic development, neural progenitor cells divide rapidly to generate a large pool of neurons and glial cells. During adulthood, neurogenesis occurs in the two main regions of the brain: the hippocampus and the olfactory bulb. In both cases, new neurons replace old, damaged or lost neurons.

Glial Cells And Their Importance

In neurobiology, glial cells (also known as glia or neuroglia) are supporting cells of the nervous system that provide structural and metabolic support for neurons. Examples of these include astrocytes, oligodendrocytes, ependymal cells, Schwann cells, and microglial cells. These cells play important roles in providing physical insulation, facilitating communication between neurons, maintaining the chemical environment of the synaptic cleft, and providing nutrition to neurons. They also play an important role in helping maintain homeostasis within the nervous system.

In addition to their supportive roles for neurons, glial cells have been shown to be active participants in information processing and learning. For example, astrocytes have been shown to contribute to learning and memory through the production of neurotransmitters such as glutamate and acetylcholine. Glial cells are also involved in modulating synaptic plasticity, which is one of the key components of learning and memory.

Overall, glial cells are essential for normal functioning of the nervous system, as they provide both structural and metabolic support for neurons, helping to maintain homeostasis. Additionally, their involvement in information processing and learning provides further evidence of the importance of these cells in neurobiology.

Synaptogenesis

Synaptogenesis is the process by which neural connections form between neurons. This process begins during embryonic development and continues throughout life, forming new connections and strengthening existing ones. Synapses are essential for the transmission of information between neurons, so synaptogenesis is important for brain function. It is believed that synaptic plasticity plays a key role in learning and memory as it allows the brain to create new neural pathways when faced with novel stimuli or tasks.

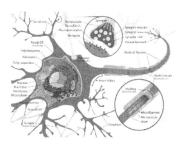

Organizing The Nervous System

The nervous system can be organized in several ways, including by structure, function, and purpose. Structurally, the nervous system is divided into two basic parts: the central nervous system (CNS), which includes the brain and spinal cord; and the peripheral nervous system (PNS), which is made up of nerves located outside of the CNS.

The Central Nervous System

The Central Nervous System is composed of the brain and spinal cord. This is where information from the peripheral nervous system (PNS) enters and is then processed, integrated, and acted upon. The CNS acts as the control centre for our bodies, allowing us to think, feel emotions, make decisions, move our muscles, and experience sensations. It also plays a role in regulating physiological functions, such as our heart rate and body temperature. The neurons of the CNS communicate with each other through electrical and chemical signals known as neurotransmission. Neurotransmitters help regulate mood, alertness, sleep-wake cycles, and many other bodily functions. The brain is composed of billions of neurons that are interconnected in an intricate network that allows us to process information and make decisions.

The Peripheral Nervous System

The Peripheral Nervous System is composed of neurons outside the brain and spinal cord, including those that control our sense organs, muscles, and glands. It is responsible for connecting the CNS to the rest of our body by transmitting sensory information from the environment to the brain and sending motor signals from the brain to our muscles. Additionally, it plays a role in gathering information about the internal environment of our body, such as temperature and body position. The PNS is divided into two parts: the somatic nervous system (SNS) and the autonomic nervous system (ANS).

The Somatic Nervous System

The Somatic Nervous System is responsible for voluntary movement. This system sends signals from the brain to our muscles, allowing us to move voluntarily in response to external stimuli. For example, when we see an object and reach out to grab it, the SNS sends motor signals from the brain to our arms and hands, which then move to grab the object.

The Autonomic Nervous System

The Autonomic Nervous System is responsible for regulating involuntary body functions, such as blood pressure and digestion. It is divided into two branches: the sympathetic nervous system and the parasympathetic nervous system. The sympathetic nervous system mediates fight-or-flight responses and increases bodily functions such as heart rate, respiration, and perspiration. The parasympathetic nervous system is responsible for calming the body down and slowing bodily processes such as digestion. It helps us to relax and restore energy after we have responded to a stimulus. Together, the two branches of the ANS work together to maintain homeostasis in the body and respond appropriately to both external and internal stimuli.

CHAPTER 4: EXPLORING THE MECHANISMS OF LEARNING AND MEMORY IN THE BRAIN

The brain is an incredibly complex organ that mediates learning and memory. Our understanding of the mechanisms underlying these processes has increased greatly over time, but there are still many questions to be answered.

One important factor in understanding how the brain processes information is activity-dependent plasticity, which refers to the ability of neurons in the brain to change their structure and function in response to stimuli. This plasticity enables the brain to reorganize and adapt to new experiences, forming new neural pathways that are essential for learning and memory.

The hippocampus is a key region of the brain involved in learning and memory formation. It has been found that neurons within the hippocampus are highly modifiable by experience, suggesting that this region plays an important role in learning and memory formation.

Neuroscientists are also exploring the molecular basis of learning and memory, looking at proteins such as CREB (cAMP response element binding protein), which is thought to be involved in increasing synaptic plasticity and influencing gene expression. By understanding the processes that govern the functioning of neurons, scientists can gain insights into how memories are stored and retrieved.

Recent advances in imaging technology have made it possible to study the structure and function of the brain in greater detail than ever before. This allows researchers to observe regions of the brain while a person is performing different tasks, giving insight into how information is processed and stored.

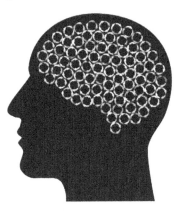

Role Of Neuroplasticity In Learning And Memory

Neuroplasticity is a term used to describe the brain's ability to change due to experiences. It is an essential factor in learning and memory, as it allows us to form new neural connections and store information for later recall. In other words, neuroplasticity refers to the physical changes that occur within the brain's neural pathways in response to learning and experience.

Research has shown that neuroplasticity can be enhanced through a variety of activities, such as physical exercise, cognitive training, and meditation. Exercise promotes the growth of new neurons in the hippocampus—the part of the brain responsible for memory formation —which helps form stronger memories over time. Similarly, cognitive training activities help improve learning abilities by strengthening the neural pathways involved in specific tasks. Meditation, on the other hand, can help reduce stress and increase focus, which can lead to increased efficiency when it comes to memorizing new concepts or facts.

The importance of neuroplasticity cannot be overstated when it comes to learning and memory. By fostering an environment where these activities are encouraged, we can help promote healthy brain development and improve learning outcomes. Additionally, by understanding how neuroplasticity works in the brain, we can better target our efforts to maximize their positive impact on learning and memory formation.

Memory Consolidation Process

The memory consolidation process is a set of events that occur in the brain to help store information for future use. It involves changes in neural pathways and biochemical processes, allowing memories to be cemented into long-term storage. During this process, neurons form new connections between themselves and become more stable so that the memory can be recalled later on. This process requires time and often involves a period of sleep to facilitate the formation of new connections.

The hippocampus is one of the main structures involved in memory consolidation. It helps store information in short-term memory, which can then be processed and transferred to long-term storage in other parts of the brain. The amygdala also helps control how memories are stored, by determining how emotional a memory is and whether it should be stored in the long-term memory.

The process of memory consolidation is complex, but understanding how it works can help us better understand our memories and learn to remember more effectively. By understanding what happens during this process, we can adjust our learning strategies and create better pathways for storing memories for future use.

Other factors, such as stress and medication, can also play a role in memory consolidation. Stress hormones can make it harder for the brain to form new connections, while some medications can interfere with the process of recall. Understanding how these factors affect the memory consolidation process is important in order to develop effective strategies for learning and storing memories. Additionally, research has been conducted into how lifestyle choices such as diet and exercise can affect memory consolidation. Studies have found that engaging in regular physical activity may improve memory recall, while diets high in fat and cholesterol can impair it.

Overall, understanding the memory consolidation process is essential to bettering our ability to learn and remember information. By identifying what parts of the brain are involved and how different factors can influence this process, we can better equip ourselves with the proper tools to help us make memories that last. With this knowledge, we can create effective strategies for improving our recall and understanding of information.

The Spinal Cord And The Autonomic Nervous System

The spinal cord is the most basic part of the central nervous system and also one of the most essential for overall functioning. It is composed of a bundle of nerves that run from the brain to other parts of the body, controlling all movement, sensation, and reflexes. The autonomic nervous system is responsible for regulating involuntary body processes such as breathing, digestion, and heart rate. It is divided into sympathetic and parasympathetic divisions, which have opposing effects on the body's processes.

Understanding how these two systems interact can help us better understand neurobiology.

For example, when a person experiences fear or excitement, the sympathetic nervous system is activated, while the parasympathetic nervous system helps to promote relaxation. This relationship between the two systems allows for emotional regulation and the formation of memory. The different parts of the spinal cord can also be used to study learning, as different pathways become activated as a person learns more information. By exploring these pathways, we can gain a better understanding of how memory is formed in the brain.

In addition to this, research into the spinal cord can help us understand diseases such as Multiple Sclerosis (MS). MS is a debilitating neurological disorder that affects the central nervous system, and understanding how the spinal cord functions could lead to better diagnosis and treatment of this condition. Similarly, research into the autonomic nervous system can help us understand conditions such as hypertension, where problems with the regulation of blood pressure are present.

Developing The Brain And Nervous System

The study of neurobiology is an important part of understanding how the brain and nervous system work to regulate behaviour, emotion, learning, and memory. By exploring the mechanisms of learning and memory in the brain, researchers can develop treatments for neurological conditions such as Alzheimer's disease. Furthermore, deeper insights into how neurons communicate may lead to advances in artificial intelligence. Scientists are also studying how the brain and nervous system develop in very young children, which can provide insight into potential interventions to improve health outcomes later in life. For example, research has shown that physical activity in early childhood is associated with improved cognitive development later on. Thus, understanding neurobiology and its effects on behaviour and cognition is essential for providing effective treatments for neurological disorders.

In addition to the study of neurobiology, scientists are also studying how the brain and nervous system develop in response to environmental factors. For example, research has demonstrated that people's brains can adapt to changes in their environment over time. This phenomenon is known as plasticity, and it implies that individuals can learn new skills or modify existing behaviours with practice. Additionally, plasticity can allow the brain to adapt to different types of stress, such as trauma, by reorganizing neural pathways. This knowledge can help inform treatments for conditions like post-traumatic stress disorder (PTSD).

Overall, the study of neurobiology is essential for understanding how the brain and nervous system work and it can help guide the development of effective treatments for neurological disorders.

Behaviour

Behaviour is an important part of neurobiology as it provides insight into how the brain works. By studying behaviour, scientists can learn about brain chemistry, neural circuitry, and even genetics. Behaviour also gives us clues about how the environment affects our brains and bodies, which in turn allows us to better understand human development and evolution. Through a combination of research methods such as electrophysiology, genetics, and imaging techniques, researchers can measure the brain's activity during different behaviour. This helps to understand how specific parts of the brain are involved in certain activities or behaviours. In addition, this understanding can also help us develop treatments for behavioural conditions such as addiction and depression. By studying neurobiology through behaviour, we gain a deeper insight into how our brains and bodies function. Understanding behaviour ultimately helps us better understand ourselves and the world around us.

Behaviour is also an important tool in understanding relationships between humans and other species. By studying animal behaviour, we can gain insight into how our closest relatives make decisions and interact with their environment. This knowledge can then be applied to our own behaviour to help us understand our impact on our planet and the other species that inhabit it. In addition, by studying animal behavior we can learn about the evolution of humans and animals and how they have adapted to survive in their respective environments. Understanding this connection between us and other species can help us better appreciate our place in the world.

Behaviour is also an important factor when it comes to mental health. By understanding how our environment and experiences shape our behaviour, we can develop better interventions for mental health conditions such as anxiety, depression, and post-traumatic stress disorder. Understanding how our brains respond to different stimuli can help us recognize when a problem is developing and address it before it becomes too severe. This type of knowledge can lead to more effective treatments that work with the individual to achieve their goals. By understanding behaviour, we can also develop preventative measures that help us live healthier and happier lives.

Emotion In Neurobiology

The field of neurobiology is expanding rapidly, and its implications for understanding emotion continue to be explored. Neurobiologists have discovered that emotions are closely linked with the body's physical responses, allowing us to better understand our emotional states in real time. Through recent studies, researchers have identified some of the brain areas involved in processing emotions. These areas are located in the prefrontal cortex, the amygdala, and other regions of the brain.

The amygdala plays a key role in emotion processing by helping to modulate our emotional reactions. It has been found that when an individual feels fear or anxiety, neurons in the amygdala are activated and can lead to increased heart rate, sweating, and other physical responses. In addition, the amygdala may also be involved in helping to control our emotional responses by regulating how we interpret and act on different emotions.

The prefrontal cortex is another important brain area that has been linked to emotion processing. This part of the brain is responsible for higher-level thinking and decision-making. Studies have shown that this region can help us regulate our emotions, allowing us to better manage our responses and behaviour in different situations.

Overall, the field of neurobiology has provided a valuable window into understanding emotion. By exploring how brain areas like the amygdala and prefrontal cortex work together to process emotion, researchers are able to gain insight into why we behave and feel the way we do. This knowledge is important for developing effective interventions for managing emotions, improving mental health, and helping us better understand both ourselves and others.

Learning

Learning is an essential process that allows us to acquire, store and recall information. Learning occurs when we interact with our environment through experience, instruction or observation. Neurobiology plays a key role in the learning process as it helps regulate our memory, attention, and decisions. Our brains are constantly taking cues from the world around us and using this information to form new neural connections which are then used to store information. Through these neural pathways, we create memories and build upon them as we experience new things. The connections created in our brains when learning can be strengthened with practice and repetition, allowing us to recall information more easily. Neurobiological research has revealed that the brain is capable of forming many different types of learning-related associations such as associative, spatial, and emotional learning. By understanding how neurobiology contributes to the learning process, we can better understand how our brains take in new information and use it to form new memories.

In addition to neurobiological research, psychological studies have also contributed greatly to our understanding of learning and memory. Psychological theories such as classical conditioning, operant conditioning, cognitive psychology, and social learning theory have provided insight into how our brains process information and form new memories. By studying the psychological theories of learning, we can gain a better understanding of how to effectively learn new information and recall it quickly.

Recent advances in technology have also opened up exciting new possibilities for understanding how we learn. Artificial intelligence (AI) and machine learning algorithms are being used to develop computer systems which can learn and remember information from experience. By using these algorithms, we can gain insight into how the brain processes new information and stores memories. This research could lead to exciting developments in education and memory retrieval technologies.

CHAPTER 5: HOW THE BRAIN WORKS AND PROCESSES INFORMATION

The brain is made up of billions of neurons, which are the basic building blocks of all neural networks. Neurons communicate with each other through electrical impulses and release chemical messengers called neurotransmitters that travel across synapses to transmit messages from one neuron to another. In this way, neurons create complex pathways that allow information to flow from one area of the brain to another. This is how the brain stores and processes information, enabling us to learn, remember, reason, plan, and make decisions.

In addition to neurons, the brain contains other cells that help regulate its functions. For example, glial cells provide structure and insulation for neurons as well as nourishment in the form of energy-providing molecules. Astrocytes are another type of glial cells that are particularly important in the regulation of neurotransmitter levels. Astrocytes act like tiny pumps, releasing and absorbing chemicals to keep neurotransmitter levels balanced.

The brain also contains specialized structures such as the hippocampus, which plays a role in memory formation and recall; the amygdala, which is responsible for emotions and fear responses; and the basal ganglia, which controls voluntary movements. All of these structures work together to help us interpret sensations, move our bodies, and generate thoughts and feelings. By understanding how the brain works, neuroscientists are able to gain insight into conditions like depression, autism spectrum disorder, Alzheimer's disease, addiction, and other neurological disorders.

The complexity of the brain means that there is still much to be learned about how it works. New research and technology continue to provide new insights into the functioning of the human brain, allowing us to better understand its structure and function. For example, recent advancements in imaging techniques have allowed researchers to view individual neurons as they communicate with each other. With further research, scientists hope to gain a better understanding of how the brain works and use this knowledge to develop treatments for neurological disorders.

These studies have also revealed a fundamental truth about the human brain: it is highly malleable and not fixed in structure. This means that through practice, training, and other interventions, we can improve our cognitive abilities and learn new behaviours. Neuroplasticity research has shown that we can rewire our brains throughout life, allowing us to modify our thoughts and behaviours. By understanding how the brain works, neuroscientists are unlocking new methods for improving cognitive functioning and treating neurological conditions.

These exciting advances in neuroscience continue to provide us with a greater understanding of the human brain and how it works. This knowledge will help improve treatments for neurological disorders and provide new ways of enhancing cognitive abilities. With a deeper understanding of the inner workings of the brain, we can unlock its potential to improve our lives and make a positive contribution to society.

The advancements in neuroscience also open up opportunities for computer scientists to create artificial neural networks inspired by the human brain. Artificial neural networks are computer programs that mimic biological neurons and are used in machine learning applications like facial recognition, natural language processing, and self-driving cars. By studying the human brain and replicating its complexity with computer programs, scientists can unlock new ways to solve complex problems.

Why It Is Important To Increase Understanding Of The Brain

The human brain is an incredibly complex machine, and understanding its structure

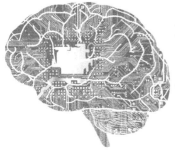 and function is of paramount importance. Neurobiology seeks to answer some of the most pertinent questions in science: What are the components that make up the brain? How do these components interact with one another to control movement, behavior, thought and emotion? By advancing our knowledge about neurobiology, we can develop treatments for neurological disorders, increase our knowledge of how the brain works, and better tailor educational approaches to promote optimal learning.

The development of neurobiology has been a major focus in medical research over the past few decades. There are now an array of technological tools that allow us to observe brain activity on the cellular level with unprecedented resolution. These methods have provided researchers with an unprecedented glimpse into the workings of the brain, giving us insight into how neurons communicate and interact to coordinate behavior.

Perhaps one of the most exciting applications of neurobiology is its potential for developing treatments to help alleviate neurological disorders. By understanding how different neural pathways are affected by a disorder, researchers can develop new medications or therapies that target specific areas of the brain.

Brain Imaging Techniques

Brain imaging techniques such as MRI, fMRI, PET and SPECT scans have been used to study the activity inside a living brain. By measuring the amount of oxygen and glucose uptake in different areas of the brain during certain tasks, researchers can get an idea of which parts of the brain are most active while performing various activities.

MRI is one of the most commonly used brain imaging techniques in neuroscience. This technique produces detailed images which can be used to study and observe changes in brain structure, activity, and blood flow. MRI scanners use powerful magnets and radio waves to generate these detailed images of the brain. These scans can provide information about tumor growths, inflammation, or any other abnormalities that may be present in the brain. They can also be used to help determine if there are any structural changes that may have taken place due to aging or injury. Additionally, MRI scans are used to evaluate and diagnose a wide range of neurological disorders such as multiple sclerosis, Alzheimer's, depression, and epilepsy. By comparing different MRI scans over time, doctors can track changes and assess treatment progress.

fMRI is a type of brain scan that uses magnetic resonance imaging to measure the amount of oxygen in different parts of the brain. This technique helps researchers to understand which areas of the brain are most active when carrying out certain tasks. By measuring changes in blood flow and oxygen levels, fMRI can provide insight into how our brains process information and respond to stimuli.

PET scans use radioactive tracers to measure the amount of glucose that is taken up by different parts of the brain. The tracers can help researchers observe which areas are working more than others, and how this activity changes as a person carries out a certain task. PET scans are often used to diagnose diseases such as Alzheimer's or Parkinson's disease, as well as to evaluate treatment progress in patients with neurological disorders.

SPECT scans use a type of radioactive imaging technique to measure the amount of blood flow in different areas of the brain. SPECT can help identify which parts of the brain are not functioning properly, and can be used to diagnose various forms of dementia or other kinds of mental illness. SPECT scans are also used to evaluate treatment progress in patients with neurological disorders.

Overall, brain imaging techniques are important tools used by neuroscientists to understand the activity and structure of the brain. These techniques help researchers observe changes in brain activity during different tasks, diagnose diseases and evaluate treatment progress. By using these imaging techniques, neuroscientists can gain an understanding of how our brains work and develop new treatments for various neurological disorders.

In recent years, brain imaging techniques have been used in combination with other methods such as genetic testing and single-cell analysis to create a more detailed picture of brain activity and structure. This kind of research can help us better understand the causes of neurological diseases, as well as how to develop new treatments for these conditions.

How It Guides You Through The Changes In Life

Neurobiology is an important tool for understanding how our brains and bodies respond to the changes that occur in life. It helps us better understand why we do certain things, like stress or anxiety. Neurobiology can help guide us as we navigate through change, whether it be a new job, a big move, or even a major health issue. By understanding what's happening in our brains and bodies, we can develop strategies to better deal with life's changes.

For example, neurobiology research shows that when we experience stress, our brains and bodies respond by releasing stress hormones like cortisol. These hormones can cause physical and mental symptoms that can be difficult to cope with, such as fatigue, headaches, or even depression. By understanding why our bodies react this way, we can better develop strategies to cope with the stress and mitigate any negative effects.

Neurobiology can also help us understand how our brains and bodies respond to positive changes in life, like pursuing a new career path or starting a family. Neurobiological research shows that when we experience positive emotions like excitement, joy, or happiness, our bodies respond by releasing dopamine and serotonin. These hormones create a feeling of well-being and can actually help us cope better with life's changes.

In addition to providing insight into how our brains and bodies respond to different situations, neurobiology also helps us understand the impact of lifestyle choices on our brain health. For instance, research shows that exercise, relaxation techniques, and a healthy diet can all help increase our mental wellbeing. By understanding the impact of lifestyle choices on our brains and bodies, we can make better decisions to ensure that our lives are as healthy and positive as possible.

Localization Of Functions In Different Brain Regions

The localization of different functions within the brain is an important concept in neurobiology.

Different regions of the brain can be responsible for controlling complex processes such as movement, emotion, cognition, and language. For example, the hippocampus is involved in memory formation and recall while the frontal lobe helps with decision-making and problem-solving.

Certain diseases and disorders are related to dysfunction within these specific brain regions. For instance, Alzheimer's Disease is a common disorder that is characterized by memory loss and cognitive decline associated with damage to the hippocampus. Parkinson's Disease is another neurological disorder that affects movement, caused by degeneration of dopamine-producing neurons in the substantia nigra of the midbrain.

The localization of functions in different brain regions makes it possible for neuroscientists and doctors to study how diseases affect the brain at a more detailed level. By understanding the relationship between brain regions and behaviour, doctors can develop better treatments for neurological disorders. Additionally, scientists are now using neuroimaging techniques such as MRI and PET scans to further investigate which areas of the brain are involved in various tasks.

The Connection Between Brain Structure And Cognitive Abilities

The connection between brain structure and cognitive abilities is an area of research that has been studied for decades. Scientists have uncovered a number of correlations between certain brain structures and cognitive performance. Some of the more prominent findings include the role of the prefrontal cortex in executive functions, such as planning and decision-making, as well as temporal lobe structures that are believed to be involved in language processing.

Studies of the hippocampus, a structure in the temporal lobe, have provided insights into memory formation and retrieval. Researchers have found that damage to the hippocampus can result in impairments in both short-term and long-term memory. Additionally, neuroimaging studies have revealed differences between individuals with strong memories and those with poor ones, suggesting that structural variations in this brain area may influence memory performance.

There is also evidence of a connection between brain structure and creativity. Studies have found that people with higher levels of creativity tend to have larger anterior cingulate cortices, an area of the brain associated with cognitive flexibility and problem-solving. Furthermore, research has suggested that certain areas in the frontal lobe are involved in creative thinking processes.

The field of neurobiology continues to uncover new information about the relationship between brain structure and cognitive abilities. As our understanding of this connection deepens, scientists may be able to develop better treatments for neurological conditions that affect cognition, as well as new strategies to enhance memory and creativity.

The Connection Between Neurobiology And Cognition

Neurobiology is a field of science that studies the functions and structures of the nervous system. It includes investigating how cells, proteins, neurons, etc., contribute to brain physiology. The study of neurobiology allows us to understand how neural circuits are organized to create behaviours and cognitive processes.

A major part of neurobiology is focusing on how different areas in the brain are wired together, and how they interact to produce a range of behaviours. Neurobiologists also strive to understand how different chemicals and hormones affect behaviour. Furthermore, they seek to understand the cellular mechanisms that underlie learning and memory formation.

The relationship between neurobiology and cognition lies in the fact that neurons transmit signals within the nervous system that enable people to perceive, process, and recall information. Neurons are connected via pathways in the brain that allow for both conscious and unconscious communication. Neurobiologists study how these neural circuits are organized such that they can produce complex behaviours and cognitive processes.

Neurobiology has also been used to explain certain mental illnesses and disorders, as well as their treatments. For example, research has shown that mental illnesses such as anxiety and depression can be caused by disruptions in neurotransmitter activity or other structural changes in the brain. This means that understanding neurobiology is essential for creating effective treatments for these disorders.

In addition, neurobiology has been used to understand how learning works, which is important for understanding how we learn skills, acquire knowledge, and store memories. Neurobiologists have studied the mechanics of memory formation and how memories are stored in the brain, as well as looking at how different types of learning occur.

Role Of Neural Networks In Learning And Memory

The study of neurobiology has provided us with invaluable insight into the way our brains process information and how it affects our cognition. Our neurons are wired together in intricate networks, allowing us to store memories and make associations between them. In order for us to learn new things or remember facts effectively, it is important that these neural pathways are firing correctly. Neurobiologists have found that our brains are highly plastic, meaning they can form new connections or strengthen existing ones throughout our lives.

The neural networks that make up our memories and learning pathways are complex and intricate. Neurobiologists have identified different types of cells in the brain which specialize in certain tasks; such as neurons for processing sensory information, motor neurons to control movement, and interneurons to coordinate signals. It is thought that these cells work together in order to form the patterns of neuronal activity necessary for us to learn and remember things effectively.

It is important to note that different types of memories will have distinct neural pathways associated with them. For example, procedural memories (such as learning how to ride a bike) require certain motor neurons to fire in a specific pattern for us to learn the skill, while declarative memories (such as remembering facts) are formed by more complex neural networks.

The field of neurobiology has advanced significantly since its inception and we now have a much better understanding of how our brains work. This knowledge can be used to improve cognition, enhance learning, and aid in the treatment of neurological disorders. As researchers continue to unravel the mysteries of neuroscience, we are slowly starting to understand the complex relationship between our neurons and cognition.

The Influence Of Neurobiology On Emotions And Decision-Making

Neuroscientists have long studied how our brains are wired and the influence of neurobiology on our emotions, behaviour and decision-making. Neurobiological processes such as hormones, neurotransmitters, and brain structure are known to shape our emotional states and influence the decisions we make.

Research suggests that emotion is an essential factor in decision-making and that it has a significant impact on how we assess risks and rewards. It is thought that our emotional reactions to situations help guide us toward the best decision for ourselves in any given situation.

It is also believed that different areas of the brain are responsible for our ability to make decisions based on emotions. The prefrontal cortex is involved in making decisions involving risk or reward. The amygdala, which processes emotional information, plays a role in assessing the potential threats or rewards of a given situation.

The influence of neurobiology on decision-making can be seen in various ways. For example, it is known that people with higher levels of serotonin are less likely to take risks than those with lower levels. Additionally, research shows that people with higher levels of dopamine are more likely to engage in risky behaviours than those with lower levels.

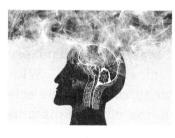

The Mind And How It Works

One of the core aspects of neurobiology is the study of how the mind works. Understanding this can help us to better understand mental illnesses, diseases, and disorders. Neuroscientists are constantly researching new ways to look at how the brain functions, and finding novel treatments for various ailments.

Mental illnesses are a broad range of conditions that affect mood, thinking, and behavior. They include various forms such as depression, anxiety disorders, schizophrenia, eating disorders, and addictive behaviours. Neurobiology offers the promise of new insights into these conditions, as it studies the brain's structure, function, and impact on behavior and cognitive functions. Neuroscientists use a variety of tools such as brain scans, genetic testing, and studying physical changes in the brain to understand the underlying causes of these mental conditions. Through this understanding, they aim to develop more effective treatments and interventions, offering hope for improved mental health care.

Neurological diseases are those that affect the brain and the central and autonomic nervous systems. In recognizing the signs and symptoms of neurological problems, you can get the most effective treatment. Parkinson's disease, Multiple sclerosis, Alzheimer's disease, and Epilepsy are examples of neurological diseases. With advancements in neurobiology, scientists are able to gain a deeper understanding of these diseases at the molecular and cellular level, allowing for more precise diagnostics and targeted treatment strategies. The development of new medications and therapies give neurologists more tools to combat these diseases, improving patient outcomes and their quality of life.

Disorders fall under another category that is closely examined in the field of neurobiology. These include behavioral disorders, developmental disorders, sensory processing disorders, and sleep disorders, among others. Behavioral disorders like ADHD (Attention Deficit Hyperactivity Disorder) and ODD (Oppositional Defiant Disorder) are often associated with challenges in self-regulation and impulse control. Developmental disorders such as Autism Spectrum Disorder and Dyslexia affect cognitive development and learning. Sensory processing disorders can affect any of the five senses and can cause hypersensitivity or hyposensitivity to sensory stimuli. Sleep disorders like insomnia and sleep apnea disrupt normal sleep patterns, posing multiple health risks. Through neurobiology, experts gain a more in-depth comprehension of these disorders, which leads to the development of more effective diagnostic tools and therapeutic strategies. This encourages a more personalized and effective approach to patient care, taking into account the individual's unique neurobiological makeup.

CHAPTER 6: INVESTIGATING NEUROLOGICAL DISORDERS AND THEIR TREATMENTS

Neurobiological research has been instrumental in discovering new treatments for neurological disorders. Scientists and physicians have used neurobiology to develop targeted therapies that can reduce symptoms, slow the progression of disease, and improve the quality of life for patients. For example, breakthroughs in understanding the physiology of Parkinson's disease have led to medications that can reduce tremors and other movement-related symptoms.

Studies of the brain and nervous system have also revealed new insights into how mental illnesses develop, progress, and can be treated. Neurobiological treatments such as deep brain stimulation and transcranial magnetic stimulation (TMS) are being used to treat depression, anxiety disorders, and other conditions. Researchers continue to explore novel approaches for using neurobiology to combat neurological disorders, including harnessing the power of stem cells to repair damaged nerve tissue and using gene therapy to target specific defective genes.

In addition, neurobiology has deepened our

understanding of how we learn and remember information, with implications for education and cognitive development. Studies have shown that regular physical activity can boost learning ability and improve memory performance, while research on brain plasticity has revealed that the brain's neural pathways can be modified, even in adulthood. Neurobiologists continue to uncover new information about how our brains work and how we can use this knowledge to stay healthy and improve learning outcomes.

Causes And Symptoms Of Amyotrophic Lateral Sclerosis

ALS is a progressive neurological disorder that affects motor neurons in the brain and spinal cord. It causes muscle weakness, problems with coordination, difficulty speaking, swallowing, and breathing. Most people with ALS experience some level of cognitive decline as well.

It is not clear what causes ALS but research suggests that it can be caused by genetic mutation or environmental factors. There is no cure for ALS, but there are treatments that can improve quality of life and slow the progression of the disease.

Causes And Symptoms Of Parkinson's Disease

Parkinson's disease is a chronic, degenerative neurological disorder that affects movement control. The symptoms typically begin gradually and worsen over time, often starting with a barely noticeable tremor in one hand.

The disease primarily stems from the loss of dopamine-producing cells in the brain, though the exact reason why these cells deteriorate remains unknown. Several factors such as genetics and environmental triggers are considered to be involved.

Symptoms of Parkinson's disease can vary from person to person but usually include tremors, slowed movement (bradykinesia), rigid muscles, impaired posture and balance, loss of automatic movements, and speech and writing changes. Currently, there is no cure for Parkinson's disease, but a variety of medications can provide dramatic relief from the symptoms.

Causes And Symptoms Of Epilepsy

Epilepsy is a neurological disorder characterized by recurrent seizures. It affects people of all ages, backgrounds, and levels of intelligence. The exact cause of epilepsy is unknown in most cases but can be attributed to genetic factors, brain injury or abnormalities, or developmental disorders.

The symptoms of epilepsy vary from person to person. Some common symptoms include loss of consciousness, convulsions and muscle spasms, staring spells, uncontrollable jerking motions of the arms and legs, changes in behavior or feelings, and temporary confusion. Treatment for epilepsy can involve medications, surgery, diet modifications, or lifestyle changes depending on the severity and type of seizure activity.

Causes And Symptoms Of Multiple Sclerosis

Multiple sclerosis is an autoimmune disorder that affects the central nervous system, including the brain, spinal cord, and optic nerves. It is believed to be caused by a combination of genetics and environmental factors.

The most common symptoms of MS include vision problems, muscle weakness, fatigue, numbness or tingling in the limbs, balance and coordination problems, bladder and bowel problems, and cognitive difficulties. There is no cure for MS; treatment focuses on managing symptoms and slowing the progression of disease. Medications such as beta interferons, glatiramer acetate, fingolimod, dimethyl fumarate are often used to reduce the number of relapses and slow the development of disability.

Causes And Symptoms Of Huntington's Disease

Huntington's disease is a progressive neurological disorder caused by a genetic mutation on chromosome 4. It affects movement, behavior, and cognitive skills. As the disease progresses, movement becomes more impaired while behavioral and cognitive problems worsen.

Common symptoms of Huntington's disease

include involuntary movements, an unsteady gait, slurred speech, difficulty in swallowing, confusion, memory loss, depression, irritability, and anxiety. There is currently no cure for HD but medications can help manage some of the symptoms. Physical therapy may also be recommended to help maintain muscle strength and coordination.

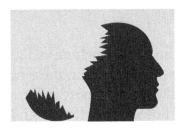

Causes And Symptoms Of Alzheimer's Disease

Alzheimer's disease is a progressive form of dementia that affects memory, thinking, language, problem-solving skills, and other aspects of cognitive function. It is the most common cause of dementia in older adults and is believed to be caused by a combination of genetic, lifestyle and environmental factors. In some cases, Alzheimer's is a hereditary disorder that can be passed on from parent to child.

Early symptoms of Alzheimer's disease include memory loss, confusion, difficulty carrying out familiar tasks, trouble understanding visual information, disorientation in time and space, and changes in mood or behavior. As the disease progresses, more severe symptoms such as loss of language skills, poor judgment, difficulty in recognizing family members and friends, and complete dependence on others for care develop. Treatment for Alzheimer's disease involves medications to help slow the progression of the disease and manage behavior problems.

Causes And Symptoms Of Stroke

Stroke occurs when blood flow to an area of the brain is blocked, causing damage to the cells in that region. It can be caused by a clot obstructing an artery or bleeding within the brain. Stroke is a leading cause of death and disability worldwide.

Common symptoms of stroke include sudden weakness or numbness on one side of the body, confusion, difficulty speaking or understanding speech, vision problems, trouble walking, and severe headache. Treatment for stroke includes medications to dissolve clots or stop bleeding, surgery to remove a clot or repair damaged vessels, rehabilitation to help patients regain lost functions, and lifestyle changes such as quitting smoking and controlling blood pressure.

Causes And Symptoms Of Migraine Headaches

Migraine headaches are recurring headaches that can be debilitating. They are often accompanied by nausea, vomiting, and sensitivity to light and sound. The exact cause is unknown but it is thought to involve a combination of environmental, genetic, and neurobiological factors.

Common symptoms of migraine include throbbing or pulsing head pain, nausea, visual disturbances (such as flashes of light or blind spots), sensitivity to light and sound, fatigue, dizziness, and increased urination. Treatment for migraines typically involves medications to stop attacks after they begin or prevent them from occurring in the first place. Lifestyle changes such as getting enough sleep and avoiding certain foods can also help reduce migraine symptoms.

Causes And Symptoms Of Tourette Syndrome

Tourette syndrome is a neurological disorder characterized by involuntary tics or sudden, rapid movements and sounds. It is believed to be caused by an imbalance of certain chemicals in the brain. Most cases are genetic, but environmental factors may also play a role.

Common symptoms of tourette syndrome include vocal tics (such as throat clearing, grunting, or barking), motor tics (such as eye blinking, head shaking, or shoulder shrugging), and repetitive movements or sounds. Treatment for tourette syndrome can involve medications to control tics and behavioral therapy to help manage symptoms. It is important to note that while some symptoms can be managed with treatment, Tourette syndrome cannot be cured.

The Potential For Neuroplasticity And Brain

Augmentation

While the causes and symptoms of common neurological disorders can be concerning, there is also potential for positive changes as a result of treatments. Neuroplasticity refers to the brain's ability to adapt and change in response to stimuli. Research into this field has led to new treatments that have helped patients with neurological conditions such as stroke, dementia, autism and Parkinson's disease.

Recent advances in neuroscience have also opened up the potential for brain augmentation. Brain-machine interfaces (BMI) can be used to restore lost functions or enhance existing ones. These technologies range from prosthetic devices that enable paralysed people to move, to implants that help improve memory or focus. Although these technologies are still in their early stages of development, they could eventually revolutionize the way we deal with neurological disorders.

In addition, researchers are exploring the use of transcranial direct current stimulation (tDCS). This technique involves applying a mild electrical current to specific parts of the brain, which can be used as a treatment for depression and other mental health conditions. It has been found that tDCS can help to reduce symptoms and promote neuroplastic changes, resulting in improved cognitive performance.

These are just a few of the ways that neuroscience is being used to explore new treatments for neurological conditions. By continuing to research and develop these technologies, we can open up a world of possibilities for treating and even potentially preventing neurological disorders.

Finally, it is important to remember that neuroscience does not just focus on the treatment of neurological disorders. It is also a field of study that explores how our brains work and develops technologies to enhance cognition, learning, and mental health. Through this research, we can gain an even deeper understanding of the human brain and its potential for growth.

Schizophrenia

Schizophrenia is a complex mental disorder that affects thinking, emotions, and behavior. It is thought to be caused by an imbalance in the brain's neurotransmitters, such as dopamine and serotonin. Symptoms of schizophrenia may include paranoia, delusions, hallucinations, disorganized speech or thought patterns, social withdrawal, and difficulty managing daily activities.

Treatment for schizophrenia usually involves medication and therapy. Antipsychotics can help ease symptoms, while cognitive behavioral therapy (CBT) or other forms of psychotherapy can help people learn to manage their illness more effectively. In addition, lifestyle changes such as stress management, exercise, and healthy eating may also be beneficial for people with schizophrenia.

It is important to note that schizophrenia is a chronic condition, and while it can be managed, it cannot be cured. With proper treatment and support from family and friends, however, people with schizophrenia can lead fulfilling lives.

Research into the underlying neurobiology of schizophrenia has been ongoing for many years. Recent advances in brain imaging techniques have allowed researchers to study the structural and functional differences in the brains of people with schizophrenia. For example, researchers have found that certain areas of the brain may be differentially activated in people with schizophrenia compared to those without it. Additionally, abnormalities in the white matter pathways and neurotransmitter systems have been implicated in the development of schizophrenia.

Researchers are also exploring how genetics play a role in schizophrenia. While there is still much to learn about the genetic basis of the disorder, it is believed that multiple genes may be involved in its development. Further research is needed to better understand how these genes interact and how they contribute to schizophrenia's onset and progression.

In addition to studying the underlying biology of schizophrenia, researchers are also looking into how environmental factors such as stress or trauma can influence the development of the disorder. It is believed that some people may be more susceptible to developing schizophrenia due to family history or other risk factors. Therefore, it is important to be aware of potential environmental triggers and seek treatment if symptoms become problematic.

CHAPTER 7: NEUROBIOLOGY TREATMENTS

P sychotherapy
Psychotherapy is a type of treatment for mental illness that focuses on alleviating symptoms and psychological distress through talking. It can help individuals to gain insight into their problems, learn coping skills, and improve relationships with others. In neurobiology, psychotherapy can be used to treat conditions such as anxiety, depression, ADHD, bipolar disorder, and addiction. Psychotherapy can be done in individual or group settings, and may be combined with medications to optimize the effectiveness of treatment. Additionally, psychotherapy can also help those dealing with trauma or grief work through their issues in a supportive environment.

Cognitive Behavioral Therapy

CBT is a type of therapy that focuses on how one's thoughts, emotions, and behaviors interact. It helps to identify patterns of thinking that lead to unhelpful behavior and then develop healthy ways to react. Research has shown that CBT can be an effective intervention in treating depression, anxiety disorders, OCD, PTSD, eating disorders, substance use disorder, and other mental health problems. It is often used in conjunction with medications to maximize outcomes. CBT interventions are often tailored to the individual's needs and can be conducted over several sessions or as a one-time intervention.

Steps Of Cognitive Behavioral Therapy (Cbt)

The steps of CBT typically involve:

- Identifying and exploring problematic thoughts, feelings, beliefs, and behaviors;
- Challenging any irrational or unhelpful thinking;
- Developing new coping skills;
- Applying these skills in the real world.

These steps can be further broken down into the following sub-steps:

- Establishing goals for treatment;
- Developing a plan to reach these goals;
- Practicing new behaviors and skills in session or at home
- Evaluating progress and making necessary changes.

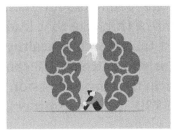

Benefits Of Cognitive Behavioral Therapy

The primary benefit of CBT is that it provides individuals with tools and strategies to help cope with their mental health issues. It helps them to identify unhelpful thought patterns and behaviors, challenge them, and learn new ways of thinking and responding. Additionally, CBT can be an effective way for individuals to gain insight into their emotions and behavior in order to make positive changes in their lives. Research has also shown that CBT can be more cost-effective than other forms of therapy. Finally, because CBT focuses on problem-solving skills rather than long-term psychotherapy, it can help individuals to become their own therapist and take the steps necessary to build healthier lives for themselves.

Limitations Of Cognitive Behavioral Therapy

Some people may find that CBT is too structured and difficult to follow, while others may find it too basic or simplistic. Additionally, as with any form of treatment, the efficacy of CBT depends on a number of factors such as motivation, dedication to the process, and individual personality traits. Furthermore, some individuals may not respond well to CBT because they need more personalized or intensive care than CBT can provide. Finally, CBT may be difficult to access in some areas due to the lack of qualified practitioners and resources.

Dialectical Behavior Therapy

Dialectical behavior therapy (DBT) is a type of psychotherapy that combines cognitive behavioral techniques with mindfulness and acceptance-based strategies to help individuals better manage their emotions and behaviors. The goal of DBT is to help individuals improve their ability to regulate their emotions, tolerate distress, and develop healthier relationships with others. It has been used successfully to treat a variety of mental health disorders such as borderline personality disorder, bipolar disorder, depression, and anxiety.

Dialectical Behavior Therapy

Dialectical behavior therapy (DBT) is an evidence-based treatment developed by Marsha Linehan in the late 1980s. It combines cognitive behavioral therapy with mindfulness techniques, which help to reduce reactivity and improve control over emotions. DBT focuses on recognizing and managing triggers that lead to unhealthy behaviors or thoughts, such as impulsiveness or anxiety. Through its four core skills modules — mindfulness, distress tolerance, emotion regulation, and interpersonal effectiveness — DBT helps clients develop self-efficacy, better communication skills, and more positive coping strategies. The goal is to help them learn how to manage their emotions better in order to make healthier decisions.

Steps Of Dialectical Behavior Therapy

The steps of DBT typically involve:

- Identifying and exploring problematic thoughts, feelings, beliefs, and behaviors;
- Developing new skills to cope with triggers;
- Enhancing communication and problem-solving skills
- Practicing mindfulness techniques to reduce reactivity.

These steps can be further broken down into the following sub-steps:

- Establishing goals for treatment;
- Developing a plan to reach these goals;
- Practicing new behaviors and skills in session or at home;
- Assessing progress and making necessary changes.

Benefits Of Dialectical Behavior Therapy

The primary benefit of DBT is that it helps individuals develop better self-awareness and skills to manage their emotions in a healthy way. It also encourages them to recognize their triggers and learn how to respond to them in a constructive manner. Additionally, research has shown that DBT can be an effective treatment for a variety of mental health issues such as depression, anxiety disorders, OCD, PTSD and substance use disorder. Finally, DBT provides individuals with the opportunity to work intensively with their therapist in order to maximize outcomes.

Limitations Of Dialectical Behavior Therapy

Some people may find that DBT is too structured and difficult to follow, while others may find it too basic or simplistic. Additionally, as with any form of treatment, the efficacy of DBT depends on a number of factors such as motivation, dedication to the process, and individual personality traits. Furthermore, some individuals may not respond well to DBT because they need more personalized or intensive care than DBT can provide. Lastly, DBT may be difficult to access in some areas due to the lack of qualified practitioners and resources.

Neurofeedback Therapy

Neurofeedback therapy is a relatively new form of psychological treatment that uses brainwave monitoring to help people learn how to regulate their own emotions, thoughts, and behaviors. It is based on the idea that the brain can be trained to improve its functioning by identifying patterns of electrical activity in the brain and providing feedback when it detects something out of balance. This may involve using auditory or visual cues, such as beeps or flashing lights, to inform the patient when they are in a "calm" state versus an "aroused" one. Neurofeedback therapy is a promising form of treatment for many mental health conditions, such as anxiety and depression, as well as ADHD and other cognitive issues. It has been shown to be effective in helping patients develop greater self-awareness, improved emotion regulation skills, and increased focus and concentration.

Steps Of Neurofeedback Therapy

The steps of neurofeedback therapy typically involve:

- Recording electrical activity in the brain;
- Setting goals for treatment
- Providing feedback to the patient about their electrical activity;
- Working with the therapist or practitioner to practice new skills and behaviors that can help regulate emotions
- Evaluating progress and adjusting goals as needed.

The goal of neurofeedback therapy is to help the patient learn how to control their own emotions, thoughts, and behaviors in order to reduce symptoms of mental illness or improve cognitive functioning. It can be a long and intensive process, but the benefits can be significant for those who are willing to put in the effort. With the right support and guidance, neurofeedback therapy can be a powerful tool in the treatment of mental health issues.

Benefits Of Neurofeedback Therapy

Neurofeedback therapy is a non-invasive form of treatment that can have significant benefits for those suffering from mental health issues. It can help reduce anxiety and depression symptoms, improve cognitive functioning, and increase self-awareness. Additionally, unlike medications, neurofeedback therapy does not have any potential side effects or addiction risks. Finally, it can be used as a tool to supplement other forms of treatment in order to maximize outcomes.

Limitations Of Neurofeedback Therapy

Although neurofeedback therapy has been found to be an effective form of treatment, it may not be suitable for everyone. It requires a great deal of commitment and dedication from the patient, as well as access to a qualified practitioner who can provide feedback and guidance throughout the process. Additionally, it may not adequately address underlying issues such as trauma or severe mental illness that are beyond its scope. Furthermore, neurofeedback therapy can be costly and time-consuming, which may limit its accessibility.

Transcranial Magnetic Stimulation

Transcranial magnetic stimulation (TMS) is a form of non-invasive brain stimulation that uses magnetic fields to stimulate areas of the brain. It has been studied as an alternative treatment for depression, anxiety, and other mental health issues that have not responded to traditional treatments such as medications or psychotherapy.

TMS works by sending electrical impulses through coils that are placed near the head, which can help to regulate brain activity and increase blood flow in targeted areas. Research has shown that TMS can be an effective treatment for some people with depression or anxiety, as well as other mental health issues such as OCD and PTSD.

Steps Of Transcranial Magnetic Stimulation

The steps of TMS typically involve:

- Meeting with a qualified practitioner;
- Placement of the TMS coil on the head;
- Setting goals for treatment;
- Turning on and adjusting the device to send electrical impulses through the coil;
- Monitoring progress and making necessary adjustments as needed.

Benefits Of Transcranial Magnetic Stimulation

The benefits of TMS include its non-invasive nature and the ability to target specific areas of the brain. It has been found to be an effective treatment for depression, anxiety, and other mental health issues that have not responded to traditional treatments such as medications or psychotherapy. Additionally, TMS does not cause any side effects or have any addiction risks.

Limitations Of Transcranial Magnetic Stimulation

Although TMS can be an effective form of treatment for some people, it is not suitable for everyone. It requires a great deal of dedication and commitment from the patient as well as access to a qualified practitioner who can provide feedback and guidance throughout the process. Additionally, it may not adequately address underlying issues such as trauma or severe mental illness that are beyond its scope. Furthermore, TMS can be expensive and time-consuming, which may limit its accessibility.

Eye Movement Desensitization And Reprocessing

Eye Movement Desensitization and Reprocessing (EMDR) is a form of psychotherapy that has been used to help people process traumatic memories or experiences. It involves recalling the traumatic event while simultaneously engaging in bilateral stimulation, such as eye movements or tapping, in order to reduce the intensity of emotions associated with the memory. Research has shown that EMDR can be an effective treatment for PTSD, as well as anxiety and depression.

Steps Of Eye Movement Desensitization And Reprocessing

The steps of EMDR typically involve:

- Meeting with a qualified therapist to discuss the traumatic event or experience;

- Engaging in bilateral stimulation, such as eye movements or tapping;
- Recalling the traumatic event while engaging in bilateral stimulation;
- Reevaluating the memory to reduce its intensity and reframe it in a more positive light;
- Monitoring progress and making necessary adjustments as needed.

Benefits Of Eye Movement Desensitization And Reprocessing

The benefits of EMDR include its ability to help people process traumatic memories and experiences without having to relive them. It has been found to be an effective treatment for PTSD, as well as anxiety and depression. Additionally, EMDR does not have any potential side effects or addiction risks.

Limitations Of Eye Movement Desensitization And Reprocessing

Although EMDR can be an effective form of treatment for some people, it may not be suitable for everyone. It requires a great deal of dedication and commitment from the patient as well as access to a qualified therapist who can provide feedback and guidance throughout the process. Additionally, it may not adequately address underlying issues such as trauma or severe mental illness that are beyond its scope. Furthermore,

EMDR can be expensive and time-consuming, which may limit its accessibility.

Alternative Treatments

In some cases, traditional treatment methods may not be able to provide a patient with the relief they need. In these scenarios, alternative treatments such as acupuncture and herbal supplements can offer a viable solution. Acupuncture works by stimulating certain points in the body that correspond to pathways of energy in the nervous system, which can help reduce pain and encourage relaxation. Herbal supplements can also be used to reduce inflammation and provide antioxidant protection from free radicals. Additionally, lifestyle changes such as exercise, yoga, and meditation can help restore balance in the nervous system and improve overall well-being. These alternative treatments can be combined with traditional medical treatments to provide a comprehensive treatment plan for neurobiology disorders.

It is important to speak with your doctor before beginning any treatment plan, as alternative treatments can have side effects and may interact with existing medications. Additionally, only a qualified practitioner should be consulted when using alternative treatments. By working together, your doctor and an experienced alternative practitioner can create a comprehensive treatment plan to best suit your needs.

No matter the approach you take, it is important to maintain a supportive environment in order to best manage neurobiology disorders. Patients should take the time to get sufficient rest, eat healthy foods, and engage in activities that promote relaxation such as yoga or tai chi. By managing stress levels and prioritizing self-care, patients can reduce symptoms of their condition and improve their overall well-being.

Ultimately, a treatment plan for neurobiology disorders should be tailored to the individual's needs. With a combination of traditional and alternative treatments, patients can find relief from their symptoms and achieve improved health overall.

Social Support

In addition to medical treatments, individuals dealing with neurological disorders can also benefit from social support. Research has shown that having a strong social support system can have positive effects on the mental and physical health of those affected by neurological conditions. Social support helps reduce levels of stress and anxiety, which in turn can help improve motor functions as well as decrease symptoms of depression. This type of support can come from family, friends, and even professionals. Those with neurological disorders need to open up to their loved ones about their condition so they can get the help they need. Professionals such as therapists and psychiatrists are trained in helping individuals cope with their conditions, and provide a safe space for them to discuss their feelings and challenges. Joining support groups, both online and offline, can also be beneficial as they provide a platform to share experiences with those who are going through similar journeys. By surrounding themselves with people who understand their struggles, individuals can find solace in knowing that they are not alone.

Self-Care

It is essential for individuals dealing with neurological conditions to practice self-care in order to manage their symptoms. Engaging in physical activities such as walking, swimming or yoga can help reduce stress and fatigue levels. Taking the time to relax and practice mindfulness techniques can be beneficial for both mental and physical well-being. Eating a balanced diet rich in vitamins and minerals also helps support neurological health while avoiding processed foods that may cause an increase in inflammation. In addition, getting adequate rest is key for those with neurological disorders as it can help reduce stress levels and allow the body time to heal. With a combination of medical treatments, social support, and self-care, individuals living with neurological conditions can begin to manage their symptoms and improve their quality of life.

Medication

Medication-based treatments are used to treat neurobiological conditions by targeting the chemical imbalances in the brain. Common medications used for this purpose include antidepressants, anti-anxiety drugs, antipsychotics, mood stabilizers, and stimulants. These medications can help reduce symptoms of depression or anxiety as well as regulate sleep patterns, improve concentration and focus, reduce impulsivity and aggression, and boost alertness. However, medications can have serious side effects such as weight gain, sleepiness or insomnia, increased risk of stroke or heart attack, sexual dysfunction or other hormonal problems, headaches and nausea.

Antidepressants

Antidepressants are a type of medication used to treat depression and other mood disorders. Common antidepressant classes include selective serotonin reuptake inhibitors (SSRIs), serotonin-norepinephrine reuptake inhibitors (SNRIs), tricyclic antidepressants, and monoamine oxidase inhibitors (MAOIs). SSRIs are the most commonly prescribed class and are generally considered to have the least amount of side effects. These medications work by increasing the availability of certain neurotransmitters in the brain, which can reduce symptoms of depression and other mood disorders.

Anti-Anxiety Drugs

Anti-anxiety medications, also known as anxiolytics, are used to reduce feelings of anxiety and panic. Common types of anti-anxiety drugs include benzodiazepines, buspirone, beta-blockers, and antidepressants. These medications work by targeting certain neurotransmitters in the brain that control fear and anxiety responses. Although these drugs can be effective in reducing anxiety, they can also have serious side effects such as drowsiness, confusion, dizziness, and impaired memory. As a result, these medications should only be used under the supervision of a healthcare provider.

Antipsychotics

Antipsychotics are medications used to treat mental disorders such as schizophrenia and bipolar disorder. These medications work by targeting the dopamine and serotonin neurotransmitters in the brain. Common antipsychotics include haloperidol, risperidone, olanzapine, quetiapine, and ziprasidone. While these medications can be effective in reducing symptoms of mental illness, they also carry risks such as increased appetite leading to weight gain and an increased risk of diabetes, and a decreased ability to think clearly.

Mood Stabilizers

Mood stabilizers are medications used to treat bipolar disorder and other mental health disorders characterized by fluctuations in mood. Common types of mood stabilizers include lithium, lamotrigine, carbamazepine, valproic acid, and antipsychotics. These medications work by targeting certain neurotransmitters in the brain that are responsible for regulating mood. Mood stabilizers can help reduce symptoms of mania and depression, as well as improve concentration and focus. However, they may also have side effects such as weight gain, sleep disturbances, nausea, dizziness, and tremors.

Stimulants

Stimulants are medications used to treat attention-deficit hyperactivity disorder (ADHD) and narcolepsy. These medications work by targeting the neurotransmitters in the brain, increasing alertness and focus. Common stimulants include amphetamines and methylphenidate (Ritalin). While these medications can be effective in reducing symptoms of ADHD, they may also have serious side effects such as anxiety, increased heart rate and blood pressure, irritability, insomnia, and loss of appetite. As a result, these medications should only be used under the supervision of a healthcare provider.

Overall, there are many forms of treatments available for neurobiological conditions. It is important to consult with a healthcare professional when considering any type of treatment in order to determine the most effective approach and minimize side effects. Additionally, many patients find that a combination of medication and psychotherapy is the most successful approach to managing their mental health.

Does Emotiv Offer Neurobiology Solutions?

Yes! EMOTIV offers advanced neurobiology solutions that combine EEG and AI technology to help you better understand your brain. Our devices provide accurate readings of the electrical activity in your brain, allowing you to track changes in concentration levels, emotional states, and even physical performance. We are also working on additional technologies such as eye-tracking and facial recognition which can be used to identify certain mental states. Our solutions are designed to help you gain insight into how your brain works and how it can be optimized for peak performance. With our advanced technology, you can unlock the secrets of your own mind and make more informed decisions about your life.

We believe in empowering individuals with the knowledge they need to make informed choices about their lives. That's why we offer a wide range of products and services including research-based solutions, personalized brain-training activities, and access to experts in the field. With our help, you can take control of your brain health and unlock your potential for greatness.

We are also committed to furthering knowledge in the field by conducting studies that explore how EEG readings can be used to understand and improve mental performance. By taking part in our research-based activities, you can help us uncover the mysteries of the human brain so that we may all benefit from this powerful technology.

CHAPTER 8: TREATMENTS OF DISEASES

P arkinson's disease

One of the most studied and well-understood neurological diseases is Parkinson's disease, which affects motor control in over seven million people worldwide. The hallmark symptoms of Parkinson's include tremors, rigidity, bradykinesia (slowness of movement), and postural instability - all caused by a lack of dopamine production in the brain.

Steps Of Parkinson's Disease Treatment

The most common treatments for Parkinson's disease, a neurological disorder characterized by movement problems, include medications, lifestyle changes and surgical procedures.

Medication is the first step in treating Parkinson's disease. These drugs can help relieve symptoms like tremors and slowness of movement. Commonly prescribed medications include levodopa (L-dopa), dopamine agonists, anticholinergics and monoamine oxidase B inhibitors.

Lifestyle changes can also make a difference in treating Parkinson's disease, including physical therapy, speech therapy, diet and exercise. Physical therapists help people with Parkinson's increase their mobility by providing special exercises designed to strengthen the muscles affected by the disorder. Speech therapists help improve communication and swallowing difficulties.

Surgery may be an option for certain patients with Parkinson's disease. Deep brain stimulation (DBS) is the most common surgical procedure used to treat Parkinson's. During this procedure, electrodes are implanted in specific parts of the brain and connected to an electrical device that helps control motor symptoms. Other surgeries used to treat Parkinson's include pallidotomy and thalamotomy.

It is important to remember that each person experiences Parkinson's disease differently, so it is best to discuss the various treatment options with a medical professional in order to find the best option for you. With the right combination of medications, lifestyle changes and other treatments, people with Parkinson's can manage their symptoms and lead

The outlook for Parkinson's patients is improving as researchers continue to make advancements in treatments and therapies. With comprehensive medical care, proper nutrition, physical activity, and stress management, people with Parkinson's can lead fulfilling lives. Hopefully, with continued research and development of new treatments, we will one day find a cure for this debilitating disease.

Multiple Sclerosis

Multiple sclerosis (MS) is an autoimmune disorder that affects the central nervous system, causing damage to the nerve cells and inflammation of the brain and spinal cord. Symptoms of MS can vary widely from person to person, but common signs include difficulty walking or speaking, blurred vision, muscle weakness, and fatigue.

Steps Of Multiple Sclerosis Treatment

The first step in Multiple Sclerosis treatment is diagnosis. Physicians use imaging tests such as magnetic resonance imaging (MRI) scans to diagnose the condition. This is followed by physical and occupational therapy, which can help improve mobility and strength as well as provide strategies to manage any pain or fatigue associated with the condition.

The second step in MS treatment is medication. Depending on the type and severity of symptoms, medications such as corticosteroids or immunomodulators are used to reduce inflammation and other complications. Drugs that target specific symptoms such as muscle spasms, bladder control, or vision issues may also be prescribed.

The third step in MS treatment is lifestyle interventions. This includes making healthy dietary changes, exercising regularly, and avoiding environmental triggers which can worsen MS symptoms. Additionally, stress management techniques such as meditation or yoga may help to improve overall well-being.

The final step in MS treatment is support. It's important to have a strong support system in place to provide emotional, social, and practical assistance. Support groups, counselling sessions, and physical activity classes are all great ways to build a sense of community among those with Multiple Sclerosis.

Overall, understanding the steps involved in Multiple Sclerosis treatment can help individuals make more informed decisions about their care. While there is no cure for MS, treatment can help to improve the quality of life and manage symptoms.

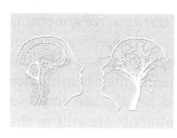

Treatments Of Alzheimer's Disease

In recent years, advances in the field of neurobiology have led to new and exciting treatments for Alzheimer's Disease. The most common treatment is cognitive rehabilitation therapy, which helps build up mental and physical skills that have been damaged by the disease. This includes activities such as memory training, problem-solving, language processing, and communication techniques. Medications can also be used to help reduce the symptoms of Alzheimer's Disease, such as memory loss and difficulty thinking. Antidepressants may be prescribed to improve mood. In some cases, medications can slow or halt the progression of the disease. Other treatments for Alzheimer's Disease include lifestyle changes that focus on diet and exercise. Eating a balanced diet and engaging in physical activity have been shown to improve overall cognitive function. Social activities can help improve memory and reduce feelings of loneliness or isolation that often accompany Alzheimer's Disease.

In addition to traditional treatments for Alzheimer's Disease, researchers are exploring new ways to manage the condition. Stem cell therapy is being studied as a way to potentially repair damaged brain cells and improve symptoms associated with Alzheimer's disease. Nutritional supplements are also being studied as a potential treatment. These supplements may help reduce inflammation, boost brain health, and improve memory. While these treatments are still in the early stages of research, they offer hope for those living with Alzheimer's Disease.

Research into alternative therapies such as acupuncture and herbal medicines is also ongoing. Studies suggest that acupuncture may be able to improve symptoms associated with Alzheimer's Disease, such as confusion and agitation. Herbal medicines such as ginkgo biloba and huperzine A are being studied to determine if they can help improve cognitive function. Although research is ongoing, these alternative treatments may offer new hope to those living with Alzheimer's Disease.

Treatments Of Huntington's Disease

Huntington's disease is a neurological disorder characterized by abnormal involuntary movements, cognitive decline, depression, and other neuropsychiatric symptoms. Treatment of Huntington's disease usually involves medications to reduce the severity of these symptoms or slow down their progression. The most commonly used drugs are tetrabenazine and xylazine, which act on dopamine receptors in the brain to reduce the intensity of involuntary movements. Other drugs, such as SSRIs, antipsychotics, and anti-seizure medications may also be used to treat various symptoms associated with Huntington's disease. Additionally, physical therapy helps improve mobility and coordination, while psychological counselling can help manage depression and anxiety. Lastly, support groups provide a platform for people with the condition to share their experiences and find comfort in the company of others. All these forms of treatment can help improve the quality of life for those who have Huntington's disease.

Treatments Of Amyotrophic Lateral Sclerosis

Neurobiology has allowed for great advances in the treatment of amyotrophic lateral sclerosis (ALS). ALS is a progressive neurodegenerative disorder that affects the motor neurons of the brain and spinal cord, resulting in muscle weakness, paralysis, and eventually death. Fortunately, recent research has enabled scientists to identify potential treatments for this debilitating disease.

One of the most promising treatments for ALS is the use of neurotrophic factors, which are proteins that help protect and repair nerve cells. These proteins have been shown to slow down the progression of ALS in both animal and human studies. Other potential treatments include stem cell therapy, gene therapy, drug therapy, and electrical stimulation.

Research has also led to the development of new types of medications that can help ease the symptoms of ALS. Some drugs, such as riluzole, have been approved by the FDA for treating ALS. Other medications are still in clinical trials and will likely be available in the near future.

Finally, physical therapy is a crucial component of ALS treatment. Physical therapists can create exercise regimes tailored to the individual patient that can help slow down muscle deterioration and improve quality of life.

Although ALS is an incurable disease, advances in neurobiology have allowed for better treatments and a longer lifespan for those living with this condition. With continued research, new treatments may soon become available which could offer even greater hope for people with ALS.

Treatments Of Tourette Syndrome

One of the most common treatments for Tourette Syndrome is cognitive-behavioural therapy. This type of therapy is used to help individuals better manage their tics and other associated symptoms. It involves teaching relaxation techniques, such as deep breathing or muscle relaxation, which can help to reduce the intensity and frequency of tics. It also helps people become more aware of their own bodies and thoughts, which can help them to better control their tics.

Medication is also used in the treatment of Tourette Syndrome. A variety of medications are available that may reduce the severity or frequency of a person's tics. It is important to note that while medication can be an effective part of managing symptoms, it does not cure Tourette Syndrome.

Other treatments for Tourette Syndrome include speech therapy, occupational therapy, and social skills training. Speech therapy can help individuals improve their ability to communicate with others by reducing stuttering or stammering that may be associated with their tics. Occupational therapy can help a person become more independent and better able to manage everyday tasks. Social skills training is also important, as it helps to educate individuals on how to interact with others in a more socially appropriate way. It can also help people better manage the anxiety and frustration that can accompany having Tourette Syndrome.

Finally, there are several alternative treatments for Tourette Syndrome available, such as hypnotherapy, acupuncture, yoga, and biofeedback. While these treatments have not been extensively studied for their effectiveness in treating Tourette Syndrome, many people have found them to help manage their symptoms. It is important to speak to a healthcare professional before trying any of these alternative treatments.

Treatments Of Autism Spectrum Disorder

One major treatment for ASD is behaviour therapy. Behaviour therapy focuses on managing behavioural challenges and improving communication, social skills, and daily living skills. Applied Behavioral Analysis (ABA) is one type of behaviour therapy that uses positive reinforcement to encourage desired behaviours. This form of therapy has been proven effective in reducing problem behaviours and increasing language and learning skills in children with ASD.

Another form of treatment is medication. Although there is no cure for autism, certain medications may help to treat symptoms associated with it such as anxiety, depression, and hyperactivity. In addition, medications may be used to control problem behaviors related to the disorder such as aggression or repetitive behavior. However, it is important to note that each individual's needs are unique and medications must be prescribed on a case-by-case basis.

Finally, complementary treatments such as dietary modifications, nutritional supplements, and sensory integration therapy may also be beneficial for people with ASD. Dietary modifications focus on eliminating foods which can have an adverse effect on behaviour or cognitive function. Nutritional supplements are used to ensure that the individual receives sufficient nutrients in order to support optimal functioning. Finally, sensory integration therapy is used to help the individual process and respond to sensations in a more organized manner.

Overall, there are many treatments available for ASD which can help improve the quality of life for individuals with this disorder. Each individual's needs must be assessed on an individual basis in order to determine what will work best for them. Additionally, it is important to have a team of professionals who can work together to ensure that the individual receives the most comprehensive, personalized care possible. By reaching out for help and support, individuals with ASD can gain greater independence and improved quality of life.

In addition to traditional treatments, there are emerging technologies such as virtual reality (VR) therapy being used to help people with autism. VR therapies are being used to help individuals with autism learn skills such as communication, social interactions, and problem-solving in a safe and supportive environment. By providing an immersive experience, these technologies can be extremely effective in helping individuals with autism gain new skills and improve existing ones.

CHAPTER 9: NEUROBIOLOGY
OF PSYCHIATRIC DISORDERS

Mental illness affects millions of people around the world, with various types of disorders. Neurobiology is an important area to study when trying to understand the underlying causes and mechanisms of psychiatric conditions. It is possible to learn about how mental illnesses manifest themselves in the brain, as well as potential treatments that could be used to alleviate symptoms. By studying the neurobiological features of these psychiatric disorders, researchers can gain insight into the biology of mental illness.

Neurobiology looks at brain structure and function to examine how neurological processes are related to behaviour and psychological states. Neurochemical systems play an important role in regulating mood and behaviour, so studying their activity can provide a better understanding of how different psychiatric conditions affect people's lives. Neuroimaging is also an important tool in understanding the underlying mechanisms of mental illness. It allows researchers to look at brain structures and activity, which can offer valuable insights into how psychiatric conditions manifest themselves in the brain.

Neurobiology has been used to study a variety

of psychiatric disorders, including anxiety, depression, addiction, bipolar disorder, PTSD, and autism spectrum disorder. By looking at how the brain is affected by these disorders, researchers are able to find potential treatments that can help alleviate symptoms. Neurobiological research has also been used to better understand social and cognitive deficits associated with mental illness, as well as the potential long-term effects of psychiatric conditions on the brain.

Overall, neurobiology is a critical part of understanding mental illness and provides an important foundation for further research into the underlying causes of psychiatric disorders. By studying the neurobiological features of these conditions, researchers are able to gain valuable insights into how they manifest themselves in the brain and identify potential treatments that could help alleviate symptoms. Research into neurobiology is essential for improving our understanding of mental illness and finding more effective ways to treat it.

Neurobiology Of Addiction

Addiction is a complex brain disorder that is correlated with changes in the reward centres of the brain. These changes involve an imbalance of neurotransmitters, which are chemicals responsible for communication between neurons in the brain. Neurotransmitter imbalances can disrupt normal functioning in areas involved in motivation, pleasure, and memory, which play key roles in addiction development and maintenance.

In the case of addiction, research has shown that initial drug exposure can cause long-term changes in brain structure and function. When someone takes drugs, dopamine is released from neurons, creating a feeling of pleasure. Over time, the brain can become accustomed to this release of dopamine and as a result, it requires more and more of the drug for the same effect to be achieved. As the brain continues to adapt, it develops tolerance for the drug and cravings for more. This is a key factor in the cycle of addiction that can be difficult to break free from.

Another important factor in addiction development is environmental triggers. This refers to external stimuli or situations that can act as reminders of past drug use and lead to increased craving for the drug. These triggers can range from certain places, activities, or even people that have been associated with past drug use and will lead to a stronger urge to use the drug again.

It is important to note that addiction is a complex brain disorder and not simply a lack of willpower. With proper help and treatment, it is possible to break free from the cycle of addiction and achieve recovery.

Treatment For Addiction

Treating addiction involves more than simply abstaining from drug use. It requires addressing the underlying factors of addiction, such as changes in brain chemistry, environmental triggers, and any co-occurring mental health disorders. This can be done with a combination of medical, psychological, and social support interventions.

Medication can be used to help restore the brain's balance of neurotransmitters and reduce cravings for drugs. Cognitive-behavioural therapy (CBT) is a type of psychotherapy that helps individuals change their behaviours related to drug use, by recognizing and understanding the thoughts and feelings that lead up to using drugs. Other forms of therapy, such as contingency management, can help individuals learn how to manage their cravings and stay focused on recovery goals.

In addition to medical treatment, individuals with addiction need to have a strong social support system. This includes loved ones, friends, family members, and other people who are willing to offer nonjudgmental encouragement and understanding during the recovery process. Social support can be a key factor in helping individuals stay motivated and focused on their recovery.

Ultimately, successful addiction treatment requires a comprehensive approach that addresses the physical, psychological, and social aspects of addiction. With the right help and support, it is possible to break free from the cycle of addiction and achieve lasting recovery.

Prevention Of Addiction

Prevention is key to reducing the prevalence of addiction. This involves implementing strategies that reduce exposure to drugs and promote healthy lifestyle choices. Education programs can be used to raise awareness about the risks associated with substance abuse, particularly among at-risk individuals such as teens. Additionally, parents need to talk openly with their children about drugs and set clear expectations from a young age.

It is also essential to practice harm reduction strategies, such as needle exchange programs and safe injection sites. These initiatives help reduce the risk of contracting infectious diseases and provide people with access to drug addiction treatment services.

Ultimately, by reducing the availability and appeal of drugs, providing education about their risks, setting clear expectations for youth, and practising harm reduction strategies, we can make progress towards reducing the prevalence of addiction.

Steps Of Neurobiology Of Addiction

The steps of the neurobiology of addiction include identifying and understanding the risk factors that can lead to addiction, such as genetics or environmental influences. It also involves studying the effects of drugs on different parts of the brain, such as the reward centres that drive addiction. This research helps inform treatments for both diagnosis and treatment, including medications and behavioural therapies. Additionally, this research helps to better understand the changes in brain chemistry associated with drug use and how those can be manipulated. Finally, researchers work to develop strategies for preventing future substance-related problems by understanding the underlying mechanisms of addiction.

Neurobiology Of Ageing

The process of ageing is marked by a gradual decline in the body's systems and functions. This includes cognitive, motor, metabolic and cardiovascular changes that can arise due to genetic or environmental factors. Neurobiological changes are particularly important aspects of ageing as they involve cellular and molecular processes that occur on a cellular level in the brain and nervous system.

Researchers have identified that neurobiological changes in ageing are associated with a decline in neuronal plasticity and a decrease in cognitive functioning. Some of the most common changes include: reduced production of new neurons, decreased activity of neurotransmitters, altered gene expression, increased oxidative stress and inflammation, and accumulation of amyloid plaques and tau tangles.

These changes can lead to an increased risk of developing neurodegenerative diseases such as Alzheimer's disease and Parkinson's disease. In addition, research has suggested that ageing is associated with structural changes in the brain including a decrease in total brain volume, thinning of the cerebral cortex and other parts of the brain, and an increase in white matter lesions.

These changes can have a profound effect on an individual's cognition, behaviour and motor skills in older age. However, there are ways to minimise the impact of these changes such as engaging in activities that promote synaptic plasticity, maintaining good nutrition and physical activity levels, and avoiding environmental toxins. Additionally, medications and treatments that target specific neurodegenerative changes can be used to mitigate the effects of ageing on the brain.

Ultimately, further research needs to be done in order to better understand the mechanisms behind neurobiological changes associated with ageing and how they relate to cognitive decline. This understanding could lead to potential treatments and interventions that could slow down or even reverse some of these changes, allowing individuals to maintain healthy cognitive functioning into their later years.

In addition, research could focus on other aspects of ageing such as the role of lifestyle factors and genetic influences in neurodegeneration. This could lead to a better understanding of how diet, exercise, stress management and genetics may play a role in slowing down or preventing age-related neuronal dysfunction and consequent cognitive decline. Furthermore, a better understanding of neurobiological changes in ageing could lead to the development of new treatments and therapies that could help individuals maintain healthy brain functioning as they age.

Neurobiology Of Anxiety

Anxiety can be caused by a number of different factors, but one of the most prominent is neurobiological. Neurobiology refers to the study of how our brain and nervous system influence our behaviour, emotions, and cognition. Understanding more about this field of research can help us better understand the causes and treatment of anxiety disorders.

The primary neurotransmitter involved in the neurobiology of anxiety is known as gamma-aminobutyric acid (GABA). GABA is responsible for regulating the levels of excitatory neurotransmitters, such as serotonin and dopamine. It acts like a brake on the system, inhibiting overactivity that can cause feelings of anxiousness. Low levels of GABA can lead to increased activity of these neurotransmitters, resulting in heightened feelings of anxiety.

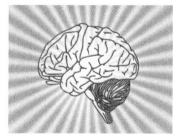

In addition to GABA, other neurotransmitters play a role in the neurobiology of anxiety. Glutamate is an excitatory neurotransmitter that plays a key role in modulating our response to stress and fear. When levels of glutamate are too high, it can lead to increased feelings of anxiousness and panic. Serotonin and norepinephrine are two other neurotransmitters that can affect anxiety levels. Low levels of serotonin may cause a decrease in the ability to cope with stress, while low levels of norepinephrine can lead to increased feelings of fear and worry.

Finally, hormones also play a role in the neurobiology of anxiety. Cortisol is a hormone that is released in response to stress and can cause feelings of anxiety. Other hormones, such as epinephrine and norepinephrine, are also involved in modulating our response to fear and stress.

Understanding how these neurotransmitters and hormones interact with one another can help us better understand the causes of anxiety disorders.

By targeting specific neurotransmitters and hormones, it is possible to treat anxiety disorders more effectively. For example, medications can be used to increase levels of GABA in order to reduce the activity of excitatory neurotransmitters and alleviate symptoms of anxiety. Additionally, cognitive behavioural therapy can also help individuals manage their anxiety by changing their thought patterns and behaviour.

Treatment For Anxiety

Once the underlying neurobiology of anxiety has been understood, treatment can be tailored to address it. In most cases, treatment should involve a combination of medication and psychotherapy. Medications such as SSRIs (selective serotonin reuptake inhibitors) are used to increase levels of serotonin in the brain and reduce symptoms of anxiety. Other medications, such as benzodiazepines, can also be used to reduce symptoms of anxiety.

Psychotherapy is another important part of treatment for anxiety disorders. Cognitive behavioural therapy (CBT) is a type of psychotherapy that focuses on changing negative thought patterns and behaviours that contribute to anxiety. Through CBT, individuals learn how to recognize the signs of anxiety and control their responses to it. Exposure therapy is a type of CBT that involves gradually exposing individuals to their triggers in order to reduce the intensity of their response.

It is important to remember that treatment for anxiety is not a one-size-fits-all approach. Different people will respond differently to different types of treatment, so it is important to work with your doctor or therapist to find the best plan for you. Additionally, it can take some time and patience to find the right combination of medication and therapy that works for you.

Neurobiology Of Autism

Autism is a complex neurological disorder that affects the development of communication, social and behavioural skills. Studies have suggested that this disorder is caused by abnormal functioning in certain regions of the brain, primarily related to language and social interaction. Neurobiological studies of individuals with autism have demonstrated differences in the structure and function of different areas of the brain. Specifically, research has identified differences in the frontal lobes, cerebellum, and temporal cortex.

The frontal lobe is responsible for executive functioning skills such as problem-solving, planning, organization and impulse control. Studies have shown that individuals with autism tend to have decreased volume of grey matter in this area of the brain compared to those without autism. This may explain why some individuals with autism struggle with executive functioning skills.

The cerebellum is responsible for coordinating and integrating movements as well as balance, posture, coordination, and motor control. Studies have found that the cerebellum of individuals with autism is often larger than normal but has fewer neurons and synapses connecting cells in different areas. This suggests that although the brain cells are present they are not connecting properly.

Finally, the temporal cortex is responsible for language and social processing. Studies have found that individuals with autism often have an enlarged temporal cortex compared to those without autism. This may contribute to difficulties in processing social cues and interpreting language.

Treatment For Autism

Given the neurobiological roots of autism, research has focused on developing treatments to target specific areas of the brain. Behavioural therapy is a common form of treatment that seeks to help individuals with autism learn new skills and behaviours as well as improve their ability to interact socially. Medications may also be used to help address certain symptoms such as anxiety or attention deficits. Finally, sensory integration therapy is a type of treatment that seeks to help individuals with autism better process sensory information.

Neurobiology Of Depression

Depression is a mental disorder that affects millions of people worldwide. It has been linked to changes in brain chemistry and can manifest itself in physical symptoms as well as psychological ones. Neurobiological research has helped to elucidate the neural mechanisms underlying depression, identifying neurochemical imbalances, genetic predispositions, and the influence of environment on mood regulation.

Neurochemical Imbalances: Neurotransmitters such as serotonin, norepinephrine, and dopamine are important for regulating mood. Low levels of these neurotransmitters can lead to depression. In addition, certain hormones, including cortisol and oxytocin, have been linked to depressed feelings. A better understanding of the relationships between these substances can help us develop more effective treatments for depression.

Genetic Predispositions: Genetics can play a role in the development of depression. Studies have identified certain genetic variants that are associated with an increased risk of developing depression. In addition, environmental factors such as stressful life events and poverty can contribute to the onset of depression in people who may be genetically predisposed to it.

Environmental Influences: Studies have found that people who experienced stressful life events or trauma are more likely to develop depression. Additionally, poverty can increase the risk of developing depression, as it is often associated with chronic stress and hardship. Understanding how the environment influences mood can help us better understand the causes of depression and how to prevent it.

Therapeutic Interventions: While the biological basis of depression is complex, there are a number of treatments that can help people manage their symptoms. Therapy such as cognitive behavioural therapy (CBT) can be effective in helping people to change their thought patterns and behaviours. Medications such as antidepressants act on neurotransmitters to improve mood. Other interventions such as mindfulness practices, exercise, and good nutrition have also been shown to reduce symptoms of depression.

The neurobiology of depression is an active area of research, and continued exploration into the biological basis of this disorder will help us develop more effective treatments and prevention strategies. In addition, understanding how the environment influences our mood can help us better manage stress and prevent the onset of depression. With further research, we can continue to improve our understanding of depression and increase access to treatments that can help people lead healthier, happier lives.

Neurobiology Of Bipolar Disorder

The neurobiology of bipolar disorder is a complex and multi-faceted field of study. Neurobiological research has identified key areas of the brain that appear to be involved in the development and maintenance of this mental health condition. These regions include parts of the prefrontal cortex, hippocampus, amygdala, nucleus accumbens, thalamus, caudate nucleus, and basal ganglia.

Some studies suggest that individuals with bipolar disorder may have structural or functional differences in these areas compared to those without the condition. This could include a decrease in grey matter volume, an increase in white matter volume, altered neurotransmitter levels, or disturbances in connectivity between different brain regions.

Furthermore, genetic factors may also play a role in the development of bipolar disorder, as certain gene variants have been found to be associated with an increased risk for this mental health condition. In addition, environmental factors such as stress or trauma can also contribute to the onset and exacerbation of symptoms in individuals with bipolar disorder.

In order to better understand and ultimately treat bipolar disorder, continued research is needed into its neurobiological underpinnings. This includes further investigations into the various brain regions and pathways involved in the disorder, as well as an exploration of its genetic and environmental components. With further advancements in this field, it may one day be possible to identify reliable biomarkers that can aid in diagnosis and provide insight into potential treatment strategies. Through a better understanding of the neurobiology of bipolar disorder, we may be able to improve outcomes and quality of life for those affected by this condition.

Treatment Considerations For Bipolar Disorder

While there is currently no cure for bipolar disorder, there are a range of treatments available that can help to reduce symptoms and manage the condition. The most common treatment approaches include medication (such as mood stabilizers, antipsychotics, and antidepressants) as well as psychotherapy.

Medication is often used to address some of the more acute symptoms of bipolar disorder, such as mania or depression. For example, mood stabilizers can help to reduce the intensity and frequency of manic episodes, while antipsychotics may be prescribed to manage psychotic symptoms that arise during mania. Antidepressants may also be used to treat symptoms of depression.

Psychotherapy, on the other hand, can help

individuals with bipolar disorder learn how to better recognize their triggers and manage their symptoms more effectively. Cognitive-behavioural therapy (CBT) is a type of psychotherapy that has been found to be especially helpful in this regard. Other types of psychotherapy can also be beneficial, such as family therapy, interpersonal and social rhythm therapy, or supportive psychotherapy.

In addition to these standard treatment approaches, lifestyle changes may also be necessary for managing symptoms of bipolar disorder. This could include creating a stable daily routine that involves regular sleep patterns, healthy diet and exercise habits, and avoiding stressful situations. Other lifestyle modifications may include participating in activities that provide a sense of purpose or connection, such as volunteering, taking classes, or connecting with friends and family.

Neurobiology Of Ptsd

PTSD is a mental health disorder that develops in response to experiencing or witnessing a traumatic event. It can have wide-ranging effects on an individual's physical and psychological well-being, including changes in the brain. By studying these changes, researchers have been able to better understand the neurobiology of PTSD.

One area of focus for research into the

neurobiology of PTSD is the possible role of the amygdala. The amygdala is a structure in the brain that has been linked to emotional memories and responses to threats. It has been found that individuals with PTSD have an increased activity in the right amygdala, which could be responsible for their heightened state of fear and anxiety even when there is no immediate danger.

In addition to changes in the amygdala, other research has found changes in the hippocampus. The hippocampus is another structure in the brain that is responsible for memory formation and recall. Studies have found that individuals with PTSD have a decreased volume of the hippocampus, which could explain why they often experience difficulty recalling memories related to a traumatic event.

These neurobiological changes can help explain some of the symptoms associated with PTSD, such as difficulty sleeping, memories of the traumatic event that are intrusive and vivid, hypervigilance, and avoidance behaviours. Research into the neurobiology of PTSD can also help inform treatments for individuals who suffer from this disorder.

One possible approach to treating PTSD is through medications that target specific brain areas or chemicals to reduce symptoms associated with the disorder. For example, medications that target serotonin pathways in the brain have been found to be effective in alleviating some of the symptoms of PTSD. In addition, cognitive-behavioural therapy (CBT) has also been found to help manage the symptoms of PTSD by helping individuals confront their traumatic memories and develop coping strategies to manage them.

Overall, research into the neurobiology of PTSD can help us to better understand the disorder and develop more effective treatments for individuals who suffer from it. With continued research, we may be able to gain a deeper understanding of the brain changes associated with PTSD and use this knowledge to create even more targeted treatments for those affected by this disorder.

Neurobiology Of Trauma

Trauma is a unique experience for every person that can have long-term effects on their physical, psychological, and social health. Research has shown that trauma can lead to changes in the structure and functioning of the brain. Neurobiological studies demonstrate the impact of trauma on various regions of the brain including the hippocampus, prefrontal cortex, and amygdala among others.

The hippocampus is involved in the formation of new memories, but research suggests that trauma can lead to hippocampal shrinkage. This shrinkage might make it harder for a person to learn new things and form new memories. It could also interfere with the functioning of the prefrontal cortex which plays an important role in decision-making, behaviour regulation and emotional processing.

The amygdala is involved in processing emotions such as fear and anxiety, and research suggests that trauma can lead to increased activity in the amygdala. This could lead to difficulty regulating emotions which in turn could make it harder for a person to effectively cope with stress. Research also suggests that hyperactivity of the amygdala can contribute to post-traumatic stress disorder (PTSD).

The research looking into the neurobiology of trauma has helped to shed light on the complex and far-reaching effects it can have. By understanding more about how trauma affects the brain, we can better support those who need it and provide them with appropriate treatment. Furthermore, this knowledge can be used to develop preventive strategies that are tailored to a person's individual experience.

While the neurobiological effects of trauma can be profound, it is important to remember that these effects are not permanent and recovery is possible. With proper support, the brain can adapt and heal from traumatic experiences. This emphasizes the power of resilience in getting through challenging times and provides hope for those affected by trauma.

Also worth noting is the connection between trauma and mental health disorders. Studies have found that traumatic experiences can lead to a greater risk of developing depression, anxiety, post-traumatic stress disorder (PTSD), and other mental health issues. People who experience trauma may also struggle with substance abuse or self-harm. People need to understand the connection between their past traumas and their current mental health, so they can seek out necessary treatments. It's also important to realize that trauma is not something one has to overcome on their own—it's possible to find help and support from family, friends, therapists or other mental health professionals. Talking with a trained professional can help people who have experienced trauma work through their pain in a healthy way, navigate their emotions, and learn to cope with the effects of trauma on their psychological well-being.

Additionally, neurobiology can play an important role in understanding how trauma affects the brain. In particular, studies suggest that traumatic experiences can cause changes in the hippocampus—the part of the brain associated with learning and memory—which may explain why some people find it difficult to recall memories of traumatic events. Other studies have also found that people who have experienced trauma may have higher levels of stress hormones, such as cortisol and adrenaline, which can lead to increased feelings of anxiety and depression. Understanding the neurobiology behind the effects of trauma can help mental health professionals better understand how to best support their clients in overcoming their trauma.

Neurobiology Of Sleep

Sleep plays a key role in the functioning of our nervous system. It helps us to restore and repair our physical health, mental well-being, and emotional stability. Sleep is also essential for proper learning and memory formation.

The processes that occur during sleep are complex; they involve multiple systems within the body including the brain, endocrine system, hormones, and motor and sensory systems.

Neurobiology studies have shown that sleep consists of two distinct states — non-rapid eye movement (NREM) and rapid eye movement (REM). NREM is primarily associated with deep, restorative sleep while REM is associated with dream activity. During the night, these two states alternate in a cyclic pattern; typically, NREM sleep occurs first and is followed by REM sleep.

It is believed that NREM and REM sleep are necessary for different aspects of our daily functioning. NREM appears to be important for the repair of physical health, while REM may be critical for the regulation of emotion and memory consolidation. During both states, numerous hormones are released as well as neurotransmitters which affect our alertness, emotional regulation, and learning.

In addition to the two distinct sleep states of NREM and REM, there are a number of phases within each state. For example, during NREM sleep there is an activation phase (when neurons fire rapidly in order to achieve a level of alertness) followed by a deactivation phase (when nerve activity is slowed down and we become more relaxed). Within REM sleep there is also an activation phase which is associated with dreaming.

The neurobiology of sleep helps to further our understanding of the importance of restorative sleep. By studying these processes, we can gain insight into how various hormones and neurotransmitters are affected by different types and phases of sleep. This knowledge can help us to better regulate our sleep patterns and address potential problems related to insomnia or other sleep disorders.

In addition, research in this area has helped to shed light on the role of sleep in various aspects of our mental health, such as its effect on mood regulation, learning, and memory formation. Further studies are needed to continue to explore the nuances of sleep and its impact on our well-being.

CHAPTER 10: THE SIDE EFFECTS OF TREATMENTS

When considering the side effects of treatments in neurobiology, it is important to understand that different treatments can have different effects on patients. Some medications may cause only minor side effects, while others may be more serious. In general, common side effects associated with treatments for neurobiological disorders include fatigue, headache, dizziness, nausea and vomiting. Other potential side effects can include abdominal pain, diarrhea, constipation, insomnia and changes in mood or behaviour.

What Are The Substances That Have Side Effects In Neurobiology?

Neurobiology is the study of the nervous system and its associated diseases, disorders, and treatments. As with any medical treatment, there are often side effects that come with certain medications or therapies. Some common substances that have been known to cause side effects in neurobiology include benzodiazepines, barbiturates, antidepressants, anticonvulsants, and antipsychotics.

Benzodiazepines

Benzodiazepines are commonly used medications

in neurobiology, primarily known for their effects on anxiety and sleep disorders. They work by enhancing the effect of the neurotransmitter gamma-aminobutyric acid (GABA) at the GABA-A receptor, resulting in sedative, hypnotic (sleep-inducing), anxiolytic (anti-anxiety), anticonvulsant, and muscle relaxant properties. However, the use of benzodiazepines is not without side effects. These can include drowsiness, confusion, dizziness, and even dependence and withdrawal symptoms with long-term use. Some individuals may also experience paradoxical reactions such as aggression or increased anxiety.

Barbiturates

Barbiturates, another class of drugs used in neurobiology, also act on the GABA receptor but in a slightly different way. They prolong the opening of the channel, enhancing the inhibitory effect of the neurotransmitter. These drugs are often used as sedatives, for seizure control, and for inducing anaesthesia in surgical procedures. However, their side effects can be severe and possibly life-threatening. These include respiratory depression, lowered heart rate, addiction, cognitive impairment, and in the worst-case scenario, fatal overdose. The risk of dependence and severe withdrawal symptoms is also high, particularly with long-term use. Therefore, these drugs are used with caution and are usually reserved for severe cases where other treatment options have been exhausted.

Antidepressants

Antidepressants are another category of substances widely used in neurobiology, chiefly for the treatment of depression and anxiety disorders. They function by altering the balance of certain chemicals in the brain, primarily serotonin, norepinephrine, and dopamine. Antidepressants come in several classes, including selective serotonin reuptake inhibitors (SSRIs), serotonin and norepinephrine reuptake inhibitors (SNRIs), tricyclic antidepressants (TCAs), and monoamine oxidase inhibitors (MAOIs).

While these medications can significantly improve the quality of life for individuals with mood disorders, they also have potential side effects. Commonly reported side effects of antidepressants include nausea, increased appetite and weight gain, loss of sexual desire and other sexual problems, fatigue and drowsiness, insomnia, dry mouth, blurred vision, and constipation. It's also important to note that abrupt discontinuation of these medications can lead to withdrawal symptoms, often referred to as 'discontinuation syndrome'. This can lead to a range of symptoms such as mood swings, dizziness, flu-like symptoms, and sleeping issues.

Anticonvulsants

Anticonvulsants are another type of drug used in neurobiology, primarily to treat seizures. These medications work by decreasing the abnormal electrical activity in the brain that causes epileptic fits. Common anticonvulsant drugs include phenytoin, carbamazepine, and valproic acid.

Like all medications, anticonvulsants also come with side effects. These can range from mild, such as dizziness, drowsiness, and headache, to more serious issues like liver failure and bone marrow suppression. It is important to follow the instructions of your doctor when taking anticonvulsants and report any unusual symptoms immediately.

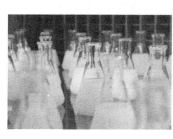

Antipsychotics

The last type of medication antipsychotics, are used primarily to treat psychotic disorders such as schizophrenia. These drugs work by altering the effects of neurotransmitters in the brain, mainly dopamine and serotonin. Commonly prescribed antipsychotics include risperidone, olanzapine, haloperidol, and quetiapine.

As with all medications, antipsychotics also come with potential side effects. These can range from mild to severe and include drowsiness, dizziness, weight gain, dry mouth, blurred vision, constipation, and muscle stiffness. Additionally, long-term use of antipsychotics has been associated with an increased risk of stroke and death in some individuals. Therefore, it is important to discuss the risks and benefits of these medications with your healthcare provider before starting any antipsychotic medication.

Minor Side Effects

The vast majority of treatments have minor side effects, but it is important to be aware of them in order to ensure that any treatment is taken safely and without any risks. Common side effects may include headaches, nausea, dizziness, fatigue or insomnia. As well as physical symptoms, patients may also experience psychological changes such as anxiety or depression due to the stresses of a medical condition or the impact of a treatment. Neurobiology can help to identify potential secondary and tertiary effects, with doctors able to assess the effect of treatments on patients' mental health as well as physical well-being. Any side effects must be taken into account when considering a course of treatment to minimise risk and maximise its effectiveness.

Headaches

Headaches can be a common side effect of many treatments, especially those involving the brain or nervous system. This is due to the disruption caused by the treatment and can range from mild to severe. Neurobiology helps to identify which treatments are likely to cause headaches and which may have minimal impact on patients. Doctors will also advise on how best to manage headaches associated with treatments, such as taking painkillers or using relaxation techniques.

Nausea

Nausea is another potential side effect of many treatments and can range from mild to severe. It is often caused by the disruption to the digestive system caused by a treatment, which may result in nausea, vomiting or stomach cramps. Neurobiology helps identify which treatments are likely to cause these symptoms, so that they can be managed accordingly. Doctors may also advise patients to take antiemetic medications or dietary changes to reduce nausea associated with treatments.

Dizziness

Dizziness is another potential side effect of some treatments and can range from mild to severe. Neurobiology helps identify which treatments are likely to cause dizziness, allowing doctors to manage the symptom accordingly. Dizziness is usually caused by a disruption in the body's balance systems, and so doctors may advise patients to take precautions such as avoiding sudden movements or taking regular breaks.

Fatigue

Fatigue is a common side effect of many treatments, especially those involving the brain or nervous system. This can be due to the disruption caused by a treatment, or to the body's response to the stress of a medical condition. Neurobiology helps to identify which treatments are likely to cause fatigue, allowing doctors to make any necessary adjustments. Patients may need to rest more frequently during a course of treatment, and medication may also be prescribed in order to help reduce fatigue associated with a particular treatment.

Insomnia

Insomnia is another potential side effect of many treatments and can range from mild to severe. Neurobiology helps identify which treatments are likely to cause insomnia, enabling doctors to manage the symptom accordingly. Patients may need to make lifestyle changes in order to reduce insomnia associated with treatments, such as avoiding caffeine or exercising regularly. Additionally, medication may be prescribed in order to help regulate sleeping patterns and reduce the severity of insomnia.

Psychological Effects

In addition to physical side effects, treatments may also cause psychological changes such as anxiety or depression. Neurobiology can help identify which treatments are likely to have an effect on mental health, allowing doctors to consider any necessary adjustments. Patients may need to find ways to manage stress associated with a course of treatment, and may also be prescribed medication in order to reduce any psychological side effects. It is important that these symptoms are taken seriously and managed accordingly, as they can have a negative impact on the patient's overall well-being.

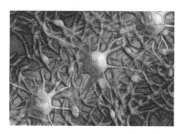

The Side Effects Of Treatments On Neurons

Positive side effects may include improved neuronal communication or increased neuron production, while negative side effects might involve decreased neuronal stimulation or impaired neural plasticity. It is important to remember that not all treatments are the same and different treatments may have different effects on neurons. Therefore, when considering any treatment option for a neurological disorder, it is important to research the type of treatment and its potential side effects on neurons. It is also important to consult a medical professional; they can provide invaluable advice about the best course of action for treating neurological disorders.

Furthermore, some treatments may involve targeting specific parts of the brain or nervous system. For example, Deep Brain Stimulation (DBS) involves surgically implanting electrodes into a specific part of the brain. This is often used to treat neurological disorders such as Parkinson's disease, but can also cause side effects such as fatigue, confusion, and headaches. It is important to be aware of these possible side effects when considering DBS as a treatment option.

In addition to treatments that target specific parts of the brain or nervous system, some drugs can be used to treat neurological disorders. Drugs such as antidepressants, antipsychotics, and anticonvulsants may have beneficial effects on neurons; however, they may also cause side effects such as blurred vision, drowsiness, and nausea. As with any treatment option, it is important to research the potential side effects of drugs before beginning any kind of treatment.

Finally, lifestyle changes can also be effective in treating neurological disorders. For example, exercise and a healthy diet may help improve the functioning of neurons by reducing inflammation and improving oxygen flow to the brain. Additionally, stress reduction techniques such as yoga or mindfulness meditation can help reduce the effects of stress hormones on neurons. Making positive lifestyle changes can often help improve neuronal functioning without the need for other treatments.

The Side Effects Of Treatments Nervous System

These may include headaches, drowsiness, confusion, coordination problems, vision problems and even seizures. In addition, certain medications used in neurological treatments may also produce other side effects such as weight gain or loss of appetite. It is important to discuss with your doctor any potential side effects of the treatment before proceeding.

It is also important to recognize that certain treatments may cause changes in the brain itself which can lead to long-term effects. For example, anticonvulsants used to treat epilepsy and other seizure disorders can increase the risk of developing depression or anxiety symptoms. Other medications such as antidepressants or antipsychotics can also affect cognitive functioning and produce lasting side effects. Therefore, it is important to be aware of the potential risks associated with any treatment plan before proceeding.

Finally, treatments that involve electrical stimulation of the brain may also produce side effects such as memory loss or confusion. The most common type of this kind of treatment is transcranial magnetic stimulation, which produces a magnetic field that affects nerve cells in the brain to help relieve certain symptoms.

Although it is a relatively safe procedure, there have been reports of confusion or memory loss as a result of the treatment. It is important to discuss any potential risks and side effects with your doctor before proceeding with this type of treatment.

It is also important to recognize that certain treatments may interact negatively with other medications. For example, antiepileptic drugs can interact with certain antidepressants, sedatives, and even some pain medications. It is important to inform your doctor of any other medications that you are taking in order to ensure the safety and efficacy of the treatment plan. Additionally, lifestyle modifications such as dietary changes or exercise may be beneficial when combined with recommended treatments for neurological conditions.

Examine The Effect Of Drugs On Neurobiology

The effects of drugs on the brain and nervous system may be divided into two distinct categories: those that affect the function of neurons, and those that act directly on cells in the nervous system. These latter types of drugs are known as psychotropic drugs, and they can include everything from simple anxiolytics to more complex mood stabilizers. An example of a drug that affects neuron function is cocaine, which binds to dopamine receptors in the brain and increases levels of this neurotransmitter, causing intense feelings of pleasure.

In addition to affecting neuronal activity, drugs can also have an effect on glial cells in the nervous system. Glia are non-neuronal cells that provide essential support for neurons by providing insulation and aiding in the rapid propagation of electrical signals. Certain drugs, such as alcohol or cannabinoids, can directly interact with these cells and alter their functions. For example, alcohol reduces the activity levels of glia, causing them to become less efficient at helping neurons propagate signals.

The effects of drugs on neurobiology are not limited to direct action on neuronal or glial cells. Drugs can also affect the production and release of neurotransmitters, which are essential for proper brain functioning. For instance, certain drugs such as benzodiazepines can increase levels of the neurotransmitter GABA, helping to reduce symptoms of anxiety and insomnia.

Finally, drugs can also affect neurobiology by altering structural components in the brain. This includes changes in the number or size of neurons or the formation of new neural pathways. For example, drugs such as ecstasy can increase the number and size of certain neurons in the brain, resulting in increased processing power and improved cognitive function.

CHAPTER 11: WHAT ARE THE TYPES OF NEUROBIOLOGY RESEARCH?

N eurobiology steps

1. Understand the basic structure and function of neurons. Neurons are cells that comprise the nervous system, and they communicate with each other through electrical signals. In order to understand how neurons interact, it is important to learn about their anatomy and physiology; such as the properties of nerve fibres, dendrites, and axons.

2. Learn about neurotransmitters, which are chemicals that facilitate communication between neurons. Neurotransmitters allow for the transmission of signals from one neuron to another.

3. Explore how the brain processes and stores information. Neurons form networks in the brain where they communicate with each other, forming memories and patterns of behaviour. Understanding these networks is essential to understanding neurobiology as a whole.

4. Study the development of the nervous system, from its early formation in the embryo to its maturation into a full-fledged organ. This is important for understanding how certain genetic disorders can affect development and behaviour.

5. Examine the effect of drugs, toxins, and injury on neurons and their functioning. For example, understand how certain medications or drugs can affect the function of neurons or how a stroke might damage certain areas of the brain.

6. Research the latest developments and advancements in neuroscience, such as deep learning and artificial intelligence. Understanding these technologies is essential to understanding how they are changing our understanding of neurobiology and its practical applications.

7. Consider the ethical implications of some of these advances in neurology. For example, the use of gene-editing technology in treating neurological disorders or the ethical considerations surrounding brain-machine interfaces that allow for direct communication between a computer and a person's brain.

8. Learn about treatments for various neurological diseases such as Alzheimer's,

Parkinson's, and stroke. Understand how these conditions affect neurons and their functioning and the available treatments that can help manage these conditions.

9. Consider the implications of neuroscience on society, such as its use in fields like education or law enforcement. It is important to understand how advances in neurobiology can shape our understanding of human behaviour and social interactions.

10. Lastly, remember that neurobiology is a rapidly changing field and new discoveries are being made every day. Stay abreast of the latest developments and consider the implications they may have for society. This will help you stay informed about this exciting and ever-changing field of study.

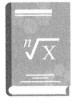

Neurobiology Current Research

Neurobiology research is an area that is rapidly growing and evolving. Scientists are constantly exploring new ways to understand the nervous system, ranging from the study of single neurons to complex brain networks.

Current projects include studying the effects of neural stem cells on recovery after a stroke or injury, understanding how particular genetic mutations can affect neuronal development and behaviour, exploring the roles of hormones and neurotransmitters in controlling neuron activity, investigating how nerve cells communicate with each other to form memories and patterns of behaviour and examining the effects of drugs, toxins, and injury on neurons.

In addition to gaining a better understanding of how the nervous system works, neurobiologists are also looking for ways to apply this knowledge in practical applications, such as developing treatments for neurological disorders like Alzheimer's or Parkinson's disease. Other areas of research include exploring new technologies such as deep learning and artificial intelligence and considering the ethical implications of using these technologies in neurology.

What Are The Types Of Neurobiology Research?

Neurobiology is an incredibly exciting field that is rapidly evolving and has many potential practical applications. Researchers are constantly making new discoveries that can help us better understand the nervous system and how it works, as well as finding ways to apply this knowledge to make our lives easier and healthier.

Neurobiology research involves studying the functioning of neurons, the cells which make up our nervous system. This type of research can take many forms, including observation of the behaviour and anatomy of animals or humans, imaging techniques such as CT scans and MRI scans, and biochemistry experiments to understand nerve cell communication at a molecular level.

One common form of neurobiology research is electrophysiology, in which electrodes are placed on the scalp of a person or animal to measure brain activity. This type of research can determine how particular areas of the brain are activated by certain stimuli and can provide insight into how our brains process information.

Another common type of research involves measuring the reactions of cells to various drugs and treatments. This type of research is used to better understand how drugs work and how diseases can be treated. In addition, this type of research can also help researchers to identify targets for new treatments and medicines.

Finally, neurobiology research often involves examining the effects of genetics on behaviour and brain functions. By studying genetic mutations or changes in gene expression between different individuals, researchers are able to identify the genetic basis for certain behaviours and conditions. This type of research can help to uncover new treatments or even cures for neurological disorders.

Behavioural Neurobiology

Behavioural neurobiology is a type of research that focuses on the behaviour of animals in response to environmental stimuli. This often involves studying how neurons interact with each other and how hormones affect behaviour. Studies may involve experiments involving drugs, electrical stimulation, or altering physiological structures such as the brain or nervous system.

Molecular Neurobiology

Molecular neurobiology is a field of study that focuses on understanding the molecular and cellular mechanisms involved in various aspects of the nervous system. This research includes studying proteins, molecules, and genes that are involved in neural development, synaptic transmission, learning and memory formation, and behaviour. Molecular neurobiologists use techniques such as genetic engineering, biochemistry, bioinformatics, and imaging to gain a better understanding of how the brain works.

Genetic Engineering

Genetic engineering is a powerful tool used by molecular neurobiologists to gain insights into the inner workings of the brain. By altering or introducing new genes, researchers can study how these changes affect behaviour and neural development in various animal models. For example, scientists have inserted a gene for fluorescent proteins into the brains of mice to track and visualize brain activity. This technique has opened up new possibilities for studying the brain and its functions.

Biochemistry

Biochemistry is a branch of neurobiology concerned with the study of how biochemical processes in cells, tissues, and organs affect the functioning of the nervous system. Researchers utilize techniques such as immunohistochemistry, electrophysiology, light microscopy, and electron microscopy to examine molecular changes that occur in different areas throughout the brain. Biochemical research can give insight into the development of diseases such as Alzheimer's, Parkinson's, and Huntington's. It can also be used to understand how hormones affect brain function or how certain drugs interact with the brain.

Immunohistochemistry

Immunohistochemistry is a technique used in neurobiology research to examine the distribution of various proteins in the brain. By labelling specific proteins with antibodies, researchers can identify which cells are expressing particular molecules and how different molecules interact with one another. Immunohistochemistry allows scientists to analyze protein expression within single neurons as well as between connected cells. This technique has been used to understand the role of certain proteins in development, neurological diseases, and synaptic plasticity.

Electrophysiology

Electrophysiology is a branch of neurobiology that uses electrical recordings to measure the activity of neurons. This technique can be used to record the action potentials generated by single cells or groups of cells in response to external stimuli. By measuring the electrical signals generated by neurons, scientists can gain insight into how neurons communicate with one another and regulate behaviour. Electrophysiology is also used to measure the activity of synapses, which are critical connections between neurons that form the basis for memory and learning.

Light Microscopy

Light microscopy is a technique used in neurobiology to observe the structure of neurons and other cells in the brain. In contrast to electron microscopy, light microscopy is a lower-resolution technique that can be used to examine large areas of tissue. Light microscopy is widely used to study the processes involved in the development, degeneration, and plasticity of the nervous system. This technique has been used to identify differences between healthy and diseased tissue, to observe the effects of drugs on neurons, and to examine the structure of synapses.

Electron Microscopy

Electron microscopy is a technique used in neurobiology research to examine structures at very high resolution. This technique utilizes electrons rather than light to form images of cells and tissues in order to resolve features that cannot be seen with light microscopy. Electron microscopy is used to study the structure of neurons, synapses, and other cellular components in order to gain insight into how these structures are organized and regulated. This technique has been used to observe the effects of drugs and disease on neuronal structure as well as to understand synaptic plasticity.

Computational Neuroscience

Computational neuroscience is a branch of neurobiology that combines theoretical and experimental approaches to study the principles of brain function. This field uses techniques from computer science, mathematics, and engineering to build models of neural systems and analyze data generated by experiments. Computational neuroscience is used to understand how neurons interact with each other, how information is processed in the brain, and how to apply this knowledge to build artificial intelligence systems.

Computer Science

Computer science is an interdisciplinary field which deals with the study of algorithms, hardware and software design, computer networks, programming languages, data structures, artificial intelligence and more. Computer science can be applied to neurobiology research as it provides theoretical models for understanding neural systems and designing experiments to observe brain function. It can also be used to analyze the large amounts of data generated in experiments, building an understanding of neural networks and brain systems. By combining computer science with traditional neurobiology research, scientists can gain a better insight into how the brain works.

Mathematics

Mathematics is essential in understanding the principles of brain function. Mathematical models can be used to describe and analyze the interactions between neurons, as well as how information is transmitted from one neuron to another. Mathematics also plays an important role in computational neuroscience by providing analytical tools for building theoretical models of neural systems and analyzing data generated by experiments. Additionally, mathematics can be used to build algorithms and computer simulations of neural systems, contributing to our understanding of the brain. Mathematics is a powerful tool for making sense of complex neurobiological data and providing insight into the inner workings of the brain.

Engineering Principles

Engineering principles are used to develop tools and instruments that can be used in neuroscience research. By combining engineering knowledge with neuroscience knowledge, researchers can design instruments for measuring brain activity, such as EEGs (electroencephalogram), fMRI (functional magnetic resonance imaging) scans, and optogenetics. These tools provide scientists with a way to study the brain non-invasively and learn more about its structure and function. Engineering techniques can also be used to develop prosthetics, implants, and other devices for restoring lost functions due to neurological disorders or diseases. Furthermore, engineering can provide solutions for building artificial intelligence systems by simulating neural networks in computers. This enables researchers to build machines that are able to think like humans and learn from experience.

By combining diverse approaches from computer science, mathematics, engineering, and neuroscience, researchers are able to gain a fuller understanding of the brain and its functioning. By studying the brain through these different disciplines, scientists can uncover new insights into neurological disorders and design better treatments for them. Furthermore, this multidisciplinary approach also enables us to build more advanced artificial intelligence systems and machines. The possibilities are endless!

Steps Of Computational Neurobiology Research

Computational neurobiology research is used to better understand how the brain and nervous system work. It involves a multi-step process that takes into account numerous factors, including anatomy, physiology, chemistry, and genetics.

The first step in computational neurobiology research is gathering data on the subject being studied. This can include obtaining MRI scans or CT scans of the brain, obtaining genetic data from samples taken, or using animal models to study behaviour. Once the data is collected, it can be used to build computational models of the brain and nervous system.

The next step in this process is analyzing the data and using it to create a model of how parts of the brain interact with each other. This can involve simulating neural networks, examining how neurotransmitters interact with neurons, or even modeling the way electrical signals move through the brain.

The final step in computational neurobiology research is interpreting the results of the models and using this information to inform further research and treatments for diseases affecting the brain and nervous system. This includes developing new drugs that target certain areas of the brain, as well as using the results to help understand why and how certain neurological diseases arise.

Overall, computational neurobiology research is a powerful tool for understanding the inner workings of our brains and nervous systems. By combining data from multiple disciplines and applying sophisticated modeling techniques, researchers can gain insight into how our brains work and use this information to develop better treatments for neurological disorders.

Bioinformatics

In addition to traditional neurobiology research, bioinformatics is a rapidly growing field of study. Bioinformatics combines the analysis of biological data with computer science and statistics to gain insights into complex systems such as the brain. Bioinformatics can be used to develop novel algorithms to better understand how genes interact and how cells respond to stimuli. Additionally, it can be used to design new treatments for neurological disorders by understanding the underlying genetic and molecular mechanisms. Bioinformatics also plays a role in developing technologies that enable scientists to analyze large amounts of biological data at an unprecedented scale. These advances allow researchers to delve into areas such as epigenetics, gene regulation, and neural development with greater accuracy than ever before.

Underlying Genetic Mechanisms

The underlying genetic mechanisms of neurobiology are complex and diverse. Scientists have identified hundreds of genes associated with neurological disorders, though the exact roles that these genes play in disease remain largely unknown. To better understand these diseases, researchers use bioinformatics to identify new gene targets for further study. Additionally, scientists are now utilizing technologies such as CRISPR-Cas9 to edit gene sequences in order to study the effects of specific genetic changes on neural development and functioning.

In recent years, scientists have also begun to explore the role of epigenetics—the study of how environmental factors such as nutrition and stress can affect gene expression—in neurobiology. Epigenetic research is becoming increasingly important as it helps us understand how environmental exposures can influence the development and progression of neurological disorders.

Neural Circuitry

Neural circuitry plays a key role in how the brain functions, so it's no surprise that it is an area of intense neurobiology research. Researchers are working to understand how neuronal cells communicate with each other via electrochemical signals along neural pathways, as well as how these pathways are organized and related to behaviour. Additionally, they are exploring how the brain forms new connections and rewires existing ones in response to experience. By understanding neurological circuitry at a deeper level, researchers can develop more effective treatments for disorders such as autism, epilepsy, and schizophrenia.

Another important area of focus is Neuromodulation, which involves the use of electrical or chemical stimulation to modify existing neural pathways and create new connections. This type of research has enabled scientists to develop treatments such as deep brain stimulation (DBS) for neurological disorders like Parkinson's disease.

Molecular Mechanisms

In addition to investigating genetic and neural circuitry, researchers are also exploring the molecular mechanisms that underlie neurobiology. By studying how proteins interact with each other within the brain, scientists can gain insights into how the nervous system processes information and regulate behaviour. This research is at the forefront of understanding neurological disorders such as Alzheimer's disease and depression, which involve complex interactions between multiple proteins. To further this field of study, researchers are utilizing advanced technologies such as single-cell sequencing to map the gene networks involved in neurological diseases. This information can then be used to develop new treatments or preventive measures that target specific molecular pathways.

Overall, neurobiology research is a rapidly evolving field that is making major strides in understanding how the brain works and identifying new treatments for neurological disorders. By combining traditional research methods with the latest advances in technology, scientists can continue to deepen our understanding of the intricate workings of the brain.

Imaging

Imaging techniques such as fMRI, PET scans, and EEGs allow molecular neurobiologists to visualize the activity of the brain in real-time. These techniques can be used to study changes in brain activity due to genetic mutations, drug therapies, and learning and memory formation. By combining imaging data with other forms of research such as genetics and biochemistry, researchers can gain a better understanding of the brain's inner workings.

Cell Biology

Cell biology is a very important field of neurobiology research. By studying the structure and function of the neurons in the brain, researchers are able to gain insight into neural networks and their role in complex behaviours. Cell biologists also study how nerve cells interact with each other and form connections to create intricate networks that allow us to think, learn, and remember. In addition, they research how neurons form and repair themselves, as well as how they respond to external stimuli. This type of research can help us understand diseases like Alzheimer's and Parkinson's, and it can inform the development of treatments for neurological disorders.

Steps Of Cell Biology Research

Neurobiology research often involves a number of steps, including observation and measurement, the collection and analysis of data, and the formulation of conclusions. Here is an overview of some common methods used in neurobiology research:

Observation And Measurement

Observations involve recording sensory input from cells or organisms to study their behaviour. This can be done by using various microscopes, imaging techniques, or other sensory recording equipment. Measurement is the process of assigning values to physical quantities such as length and time. This is used to collect data points about a particular organism or cell.

Data Collection And Analysis

Once observations and measurements have been made, researchers must organize their data in order to draw meaningful conclusions. Data can be collected and analyzed using statistics, computer programs, or other methods of data analysis.

Modeling

Modeling involves creating a mathematical or computer simulation of a particular system or process in order to better understand it. This is often done in the context of neurobiology research to gain insight into how various processes work in the brain.

Experimentation

Experiments are used to test hypotheses and draw conclusions about a particular phenomenon. This is often done in the context of animal testing, but can also be conducted with cells or other model organisms. Experiments require careful planning and execution to ensure that accurate results are obtained.

Interdisciplinary Approach

Neurobiology research often involves collaboration between scientists from different disciplines. Researchers may work together to combine their knowledge and skills in order to gain a comprehensive understanding of the brain. This type of interdisciplinary approach is necessary for many areas of modern neuroscience research.

Interpretation And Synthesis

Once observations, measurements, models, experiments, and collaborations have been conducted, researchers must interpret their findings and synthesize them into meaningful conclusions. This is often done through the use of mathematical equations or statistical models. Additionally, researchers must communicate their results clearly and concisely so that they may be understood by other scientists.

These are just some of the many steps involved in neurobiology research; however, each research project is unique and may involve different steps. Researchers need to be well-versed in the techniques used in their particular field of study so that they can carry out effective and meaningful research.

Neuroimaging

Neuroimaging is an important tool for neurobiology research that allows scientists to observe brain activity in living organisms. This research can include studying brain development in children or looking at changes in the brain caused by neurological diseases. Neuroimaging studies often involve techniques such as MRI, PET scans, and CT scans.

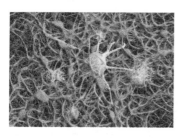

Cognitive Neurobiology

Cognitive neurobiology is a type of research that looks at how different parts of the brain process information to produce behaviour. This involves studying the relationships between neurons, hormones, and other molecules that affect behaviour. Cognitive neurobiology also looks at how memories are formed and stored in the brain, as well as how different parts of the brain interact to create conscious experiences.

Steps Of Cognitive Neurobiology Research

The process of cognitive neurobiology research involves several steps. First, researchers collect data on brain activity during the task or experiment, typically by using EEG (electroencephalography) or fMRI (functional magnetic resonance imaging). Next, they analyze the data to determine which areas of the brain are active when performing a given task or experiment. Finally, they draw conclusions from the data to better understand how the brain works and why certain behaviours occur.

The findings of cognitive neurobiology research can be used in a variety of ways. For example, it can help explain certain mental health disorders by identifying differences in brain structure or activity between those with and without a disorder. It can also be used to identify potential targets for drug development, as well as ways to enhance cognitive performance in areas such as memory and learning. Finally, it can help us better understand the underlying causes of certain diseases or conditions, which may lead to more effective treatments or therapies.

Clinical Neurobiology

Clinical neurobiology involves the study of neurological disorders such as Alzheimer's disease, stroke, Parkinson's disease, autism spectrum disorder, traumatic brain injury, multiple sclerosis, epilepsy and Huntington's disease. Research at this level focuses on understanding the symptoms of these diseases, their causes and possible treatments. Clinical neurobiology also involves the study of how these conditions have an impact on a person's quality of life and how best to manage their symptoms

Steps Of Clinical Neurobiology Research

Clinical neurobiology research involves a variety of steps, from data gathering to analysis. First, researchers collect data about the brain and behaviour through various test procedures. This can include EEGs (electroencephalogram), MRI scans, or behavioural tests such as measures of cognitive function or emotion-regulation tasks. Researchers may also use biological samples such as blood, saliva, or cerebrospinal fluid.

Second, researchers analyze the data to gain insight into aspects such as brain structure and function, disease processes, or genetic factors that affect behaviour. This can involve various types of statistical analysis, including machine learning algorithms. Third, researchers interpret their findings and share them with other scientists and medical professionals in journals or presentations.

Finally, researchers may use the results of their research to develop new treatments or interventions for diseases or neurological disorders. For example, a study of Parkinson's Disease might lead to the development of a new drug that could help control the progression of the disease. Ultimately, clinical neurobiology research has great potential to improve our understanding and treatment of neurological disorders.

Developmental Neurobiology

Developmental neurobiology, also known as developmental neuroscience or neurodevelopmental research, investigates the development of the nervous system from embryonic stages to adulthood. This type of research spans disciplines such as genetics, cell biology and developmental psychology. Examples of findings in this area include the role played by genes in neural development and how the environment can influence brain structure and function. Additionally, researchers explore the role of the nervous system in learning and memory.

Steps Of Developmental Neurobiology

The development of the nervous system is divided into three distinct stages: neurogenesis, neuronal migration and differentiation, and synaptogenesis. Neurogenesis is the formation of nerve cells (neurons) from stem cells found in the embryonic stage. Neuronal migration and differentiation involve the movement of neurons to their final destination in the brain or spinal cord, as well as the alteration of their shapes and functions. Finally, synaptogenesis is the formation and strengthening of connections between neurons, which is essential for the transmission of signals in the brain.

CONCLUSION

Neurons, often referred to as nerve cells, are fundamental components of the nervous system. They are specialized to transmit information throughout the body. Structurally, a typical neuron comprises the cell body, dendrites, and an axon. The cell body, or soma, contains the nucleus and other organelles vital for the neuron's functionality. Dendrites, branching off the cell body, receive signals from other neurons and transmit them towards the cell body. The axon, an elongated projection, carries electrical impulses away from the cell body towards other neurons or muscles. Functionally, neurons communicate via these electrical impulses, known as action potentials, which propagate along the axon. This neural communication forms the basis of all cognitive and bodily functions.

Key concepts in neurobiology are fundamental to understanding how the brain works and processes information. One of the most important concepts is that of neural networks, which refers to the interconnected neurons in the brain and how they transmit signals between them. Another key concept is membrane potential, which is the difference in electrical charge inside versus outside of a neuron's cell membrane; this can be used to determine when a neuron fires. Neurotransmission is also an important concept, as it refers to the signals and chemicals that are sent between neurons in order to communicate with each other. Finally, synaptic plasticity is a central concept when discussing learning and memory, as this refers to how synaptic connections can be modified based on experience or environmental stimuli. All of these concepts are essential for understanding the brain's functionality and how it processes information.

Neuronal signaling is another key concept in neurobiology, as this refers to the electrical signals that neurons generate when they are activated. This signal can be used to trigger changes in other cells or tissue, or even influence behaviour and thought processes. Neurons can also communicate via chemical messengers such as neurotransmitters, which are released in response to certain stimuli and can then travel across the synapse between two neurons. This type of signaling plays a crucial role in regulating emotion, memory, learning, and much more.

Finally, neurogenesis is another important concept when discussing neuroscience. This refers to the process by which new neurons are formed in the brain; this occurs during development, but can also happen in adulthood as well. Neurogenesis is important for understanding learning, memory formation, and the ability to form new connections between neurons. A deeper understanding of neurobiology requires knowledge of these key concepts and how they interact with each other to form a functioning brain.

Neurological disorders can be caused by a variety of factors, including genetic mutations, environmental factors such as toxins or viruses, and degenerative diseases. Common symptoms of neurological disorders include physical difficulties (such as tremors, paralysis, and impaired coordination), mental impairments (such as memory loss or confusion), and changes in mood or behaviour (such as depression, aggression, or difficulty concentrating).

Diagnosis of neurological disorders often involves a combination of medical history review, physical and cognitive tests, imaging scans such as an MRI or CT scan, and laboratory testing. Treatment options can vary widely depending on the cause and type of disorder. Common treatments include medications, therapies (such as speech therapy or physical therapy), surgery, and lifestyle modifications.

Individuals with neurological disorders must consult their doctor for an accurate diagnosis and to discuss the best treatment plan for them. Understanding the cause of the disorder can help individuals manage their symptoms better and make informed decisions about their care.

Living with a neurological disorder can be

challenging, but many resources and strategies can help. Some helpful strategies include seeking out support from family and friends, participating in therapy to learn how to manage symptoms, avoiding triggers or stressors that may worsen symptoms, and maintaining a healthy lifestyle with adequate sleep, exercise, and nutrition.

It is also important for those affected by neurological disorders to be informed about their condition and to keep up with the latest treatments and research. Joining support groups or talking to other individuals with similar conditions can provide helpful advice, understanding, and comfort.

Finally, individuals with neurological disorders need to take care of their mental health in order to manage stress and cope with any difficulties they may experience. This could involve participating in activities that bring joy, engaging in self-care practices such as meditation or yoga, and speaking with a mental health professional if needed. By taking care of one's mental health, individuals can better manage symptoms and live a fulfilling life despite their neurological disorder.

MAY I ASK YOU FOR A
SMALL FAVOR?

Before you go, please I need your assistance! In case you like this book, might you be able to please share your opinion on Amazon and compose a legit review? It will take only one moment for you, yet be an extraordinary favour for me. Since I'm not a famous writer and I don't have a large distributing organization supporting me. I read each and every review and hop around with happiness like a little child each time my audience remarks on my books and gives me their fair criticism! ☺. In case you didn't appreciate the book or had an issue with it, kindly get in touch with me via email D.beckology@gmail.com and reveal to me how I can improve it.

Made in the USA
Monee, IL
28 December 2024